D1288342

Work & Illness

Work & Illness

THE CANCER PATIENT

EDITED BY
Ivan Barofsky

PRAEGER

New York
Westport, Connecticut
London

QZ
200
W924
1989

Copyright Acknowledgments

The following material is reproduced with the permission of the respective publishers:

Figures 1.1, 1.2, and 6.1, from *Research in Organizational Behavior*, published by JAI Press; Table 6.1, from *Journal of Clinical Oncology, 4*, 806, 1986, published by Grune and Stratton, Inc.; and portions of Chapter 3, from *Journal of Chronic Diseases, 39*, 751–759, 1986, published by Pergamon Press.

Chapters 4 and 5, which amplify materials originally published in *Cancer, 57*, 190–193, and ibid., *58*, 2355–2361 (1986), respectively, are used with the permission of Lippincott Publishers.

Library of Congress Cataloging-in-Publication Data

Work & Illness.

Includes indexes.
1. Cancer—Patients—Employment.   2. Cancer—Social aspects.   3. Cancer—Economic aspects.   I. Barofsky, Ivan.
RA645.C3W67   1989   362.1'96994   88–25544
ISBN 0–275–92390–8 (alk. paper)

Copyright © 1989 by Ivan Barofsky

All rights reserved. No portion of this book may be reproduced, by any process or technique, without the express written consent of the publisher.

Library of Congress Catalog Card Number: 88-25544
ISBN: 0–275–92390–8

First published in 1989

Praeger Publishers, One Madison Avenue, New York, NY   10010
A division of Greenwood Press, Inc.

Printed in the United States of America

The paper used in this book complies with the Permanent Paper Standard issued by the National Information Standards Organization (Z39.48–1984).

10   9   8   7   6   5   4   3   2   1

To Chris Marshall and Helen Hartman, two patients
whose experiences initiated the editor's interest
in chronicling the effect of cancer on work history,

and

to Anna-Lisa Barofsky,
whose life made it a personal experience

Contents

Preface

You hear about it every day, in the newspapers and on television. Congress has even declared its occurrence to be unjust (Biaggi 1986). We refer to the claim of persons that they have been dismissed from their jobs, or have received fewer benefits than their co-workers simply because they have or have had a particular disease. Recently the experiences of AIDS patients have been reported most extensively in the news media, but in fact it is an experience patients with all types of chronic disease have had. Are such claims true? Were the patients victims of job discrimination or will persons without the disease have the same experience? In what way has a person's illness become part of the "normal" activity of discriminating between competent and noncompetent workers? How do we define job discrimination, and if it occurs what do we do about it?

The purpose of this book is to start to answer these and related questions for the cancer patient. The book is divided into two major sections; the first reviews the available data on the work history of the cancer patient, the second makes specific recommendations concerning future research and policy issues.

Job discrimination of the cancer patient is ordinarily inferred from self-reported work histories (McKenna 1973), or efforts to achieve legal redress. It has never been possible to operationalize job discrimination of the cancer patient by referring to what would be expected for the population as a whole. Thus, while it would be expected that a company employ the same proportion of women, minorities, and older people found in the population, this has not been possible to do for the cancer patient primarily because of the difficulty of estimating the prevalence of cancer patients in the population. The absence of a clear actuarial benchmark to use to define when a company has or has not discriminated, has stimulated the development of alternative policy approaches.

It may be useful to state, at the outset, that the argument about whether the cancer patient is an object of discrimination is a moot one, since its occurrence is an inevitable consequence of our social system and the characteristics of the disease. This statement is based on the premise that discrimination is an ordinary aspect of social processes, including work. Promotions, distribution of bonuses, salaries, job assignments, and so on, are all based on someone making a decision about the comparable worth of workers—in discriminating between workers. When a worker's physical or disease status becomes part of the decision-making process, then a type of discrimination can occur that is considered socially and politically unacceptable. To protect the worker, society has set legal definitions of unwarranted discrimination and provided a mechanism for legal redress (e.g., the Rehabilitation Act of 1973).

There are at least three ways by which the cancer patient unavoidably becomes a victim of job discrimination. First, the wage/benefit system which is prevalent in our society couples the "usefulness" of the employee to the benefits he or she receives, even though the disease the person may have requires the same financial commitment. As a result, the least valued worker is least likely to continue to be employed, receive medical benefits, or both, and a history of cancer increases the chances that this differential treatment will occur.

Second, the actuarial foundation of the social insurance system also makes it inevitable that the person with cancer will be discriminated against, since eliminating a cancer patient (or persons with other diseases for that matter) protects the larger group from the risk of increased costs. This type of discrimination is unavoidable unless the system is government supported.

Third, some patients with different types of cancer are more likely not to survive than others; some require more costly medical care than others; and so on. These differences can also become part of the process whereby decisions are made about the patient as employee, his or her present insurability and future risk of disease recurrence. Combine these factors with the circumstances surrounding job dynamics (job selection, advancement, and termination) and interpersonal relationships and the opportunities for job discrimination increase enormously.

While the opportunities may exist, there are also social factors (public opinion, statutory limitations) which would ordinarily mitigate against the occurrence of job discrimination. Thus, the empirical question remains, as does the question of why it would occur, and if it occurs more frequently than what would be expected for persons without a manifest illness.

Two researchers, Robert McKenna and Frances Feldman, must be acknowledged as the persons most responsible for demonstrating the importance of the field. To the rest of us belong the tasks of filling in, expanding, and clarifying what these two investigators originally observed and reported. They have the right to feel proud for having initiated the efforts that have matured into an increasingly vital area of research dealing with a major quality of life domain of the cancer patient.

It is hoped that the reader will come away from this book with the impression that, while a lot is known, a lot more will be learned in the future as this special topic is integrated into the larger set of studies dealing with the sociology and social psychology of discrimination, how to maximize human productivity, and how to relate these data to the formation of public policy for the chronically ill.

REFERENCES

Biaggi, M. Press release dated Sept. 30, 1987, entitled "Senate Joins House in Vote Affirming Rights of Cancer Survivors to Employment."

McKenna, R. J. *Analysis of case histories: Re-employment problems of the recovered cancer patient.* San Francisco, American Cancer Society, California Division, Inc., 1973.

I

Background Data

1

Work: Issues and Concepts

Ivan Barofsky

INTRODUCTION

Interest in studies of job discrimination of work-able cancer patients can be stated to have formally started with McKenna's (1973) report summarizing the experiences of his patients and the issuing of a request for research proposals (RFP) by the National Cancer Institute entitled "Modification of Employment of Work-Able Cancer Patients" (1973). The RFP was to have three phases; first, the magnitude of discrimination against work-able cancer patients was to be estimated on a national sample. If found to be a problem, then second and third phases were to be implemented, consisting of an action program designed to modify discriminatory hiring practices and an evaluation of this effort. These two events coincided with the establishment of the rehabilitation program at the National Cancer Institute (National Cancer Rehabilitation Planning Conference, June, 1973) and the passage of the Rehabilitation Act of 1973. Each of these events contributed to the development of a Zeitgeist that made studies of job discrimination both feasible and an appropriate response to a problem that some felt as a social imperative.

As a result of these activities, the work history of the cancer patient has become the subject of a continuing series of studies, some of which are summarized in the chapters of this book. This chapter has two purposes: first, to provide an appropriate informational background to the topic of job discrimination of the cancer patient, and second, to set the stage for the generation of a new research agenda which will integrate what is known

Table 1.1
Dimensions of Work

Analytical Perspectives:	Economic Sociological Psychological
Components:	Wages Benefits
States:	Working Unemployment Retirement
Transitions:	Job Establishment Job Termination
Pathology:	Work-induced Illness (Stress) Occupational Hazards Impact of Illness on Work

Source: Compiled by the author.

about job discrimination of the cancer patient into the well established research literature dealing with labor market economics and the psychology and sociology of work. A chapter dealing with the research agenda and another dealing with policy objectives conclude the book.

DIMENSIONS OF WORK

As illustrated in Table 1.1, work is a complex variable which may be approached from a number of analytical perspectives (economic, sociological, psychological), consists of a number of distinct components (such as wages and benefits), covers a number of independent states (working, unemployment, retirement), involves a number of identifiable transition processes (job establishment, job termination), involves evaluative activities (performance appraisal, occupational competence), and can be related to a number of pathological conditions (work-induced illness [stress], occupational hazards, impact of illness on work).

Work is clearly a major covariate of general well-being and life satisfaction for the general population (Bergermaier, Borg, and Champoux 1984; Campbell 1981). It remains a central determinant of well-being until the presence of frank illness. Describing this transition is one way to state the task of those interested in understanding the determinants of job discrimination of the chronically ill.

Work may be defined as that form of productive activity in which the individual receives financial compensation. Other forms of activities which have a productive component include being a volunteer, home maintainer, care giver, student, friend, or family member. Participating in organizations, religious activities, or hobbies reflects more individual interests and values with a less visible (economic) social product.

Each of these activities, or roles, can be scaled along a social metric in which the proportion of tangible consequences (such as being paid) or nontangible consequences of the particular activity differ. For example, most people work for money (a tangible reward) but also gain a sense of personal satisfaction from the job (a nontangible reward). For leisure activities, such as a hobby, the consequences will ordinarily be nontangible but can have a tangible component (i.e., an individual can discover that he or she can sell the products he or she enjoys making as a hobby). Those activities which predominantly produce tangible consequences are defined as productive activities.

An individual ordinarily engages in a composite of such activities. Thus, a person may work full-time, be a part-time student, have a family, and contribute to the care of the house. Describing the dynamics and shifts in these activities as a function of such factors as developmental stage (e.g., adolescence, adulthood, retirement, etc.), or illness is required for an adequate work history. The outcome of such processes would be the emergence of work-related competencies. Describing such changes in activities or roles, as a function of type of cancer, or stage in the natural history of cancer and its treatment, although obvious, has not been adequately done.

Since the number of activities an individual can engage in at any one time is limited, it can be viewed as a resource whose distribution will vary, and whose elements will require conservation. Economists have been particularly interested in the management of limited resources in general, and of labor in particular. Two conceptual approaches are particularly relevant to this discussion: the commodity and human resources (Ginzberg 1976) approaches. Our interest here is limited to determining the role of the cancer patient in the labor force and labor market, and how cancer may effect the productivity of the patient.

In the commodity model work, housework, voluntary activities, and so on, are all involved in the efforts of individuals to minimize their costs and maximize their benefits. The application of this utility-maximization model is best understood by the study of the marketplace. In the marketplace people are assumed to pursue rationally their own interests in a competitive and fluid market. Workers invest, through education and training, in their "human capital," while employers adjust wages and recruitment patterns to achieve maximum efficiency in productivity. In this world of perfect competition all workers and all employers interact, with the law of supply and demand governing levels of wages and productivity. Thus, the commodity model states that the laws that govern the economics of products also apply to the labor (or pattern of activities) of people.

An alternative, the human resources model, states that man's values and goals provides a framework that structures the activities a person engages in and that these values and goals have to be made explicit if the society is to be fair and just. The model rejects the notion that economic behavior can be described in valueless terms, and that the operation of the market model can be justified as reflecting the operation of natural (rational) law. Rather it states that consensual values and goals can structure and direct how the market operates.

The human resources model asserts that there is a profound affiliative component to economic behavior that limits the applicability of the market model. For example, the market model assumes that work is a disutility, an activity that men and women prefer to avoid, but must engage in if they are to obtain the necessities of life. In contrast, the human resources model, while acknowledging that man may want to avoid work, also states that it can be satisfying and a determinant of individual decision making. Thus, there is value in the process of work, not just the outcome of work (productivity) that determines its occurrence.

The contrasts in these two models, in many ways, capture the essence of the struggle that is addressed by an employer as he tries to make decisions concerning the employment of the cancer patient. If people, some of whom will have cancer and be work-able, are viewed as a commodity, then they should be subject to market rules. Any limitation or change in productivity in an otherwise work-able person would force the employer to minimize his costs by removing such persons from his employ. In contrast, if a person who may have cancer is seen as a potential and actual resource to be fostered, developed, and used, then the employer will want to retain and utilize such an individual. Retaining such a person may involve the cost of relocating or retraining the individual, or filling the person's position temporarily with another employee. What is not known is whether employers ever determine if the cost of such efforts are offset by enhanced organizational morale and employee well-being. In addition, very little is known about when and how cancer becomes part of the employer's decision making about his employees. It is the conflict between these perspectives, or more accurately the lack of a political consensus of what the social values should be in this context, that is probably why job discrimination of cancer patients continues to be reported.

Hall (1986) has defined work as that "effort or activity of an individual performed for the purpose of providing goods or services of value to others: it is also considered to be work by the individual so involved" (p. 13). This definition overlaps with the one provided above in that both define work as an activity which has a major social component, but differs in that it permits the individual to define the activity previously labeled productive. Hall's argument here is that an individual ordinarily defines reality based on a continuing personal negotiation, or social interaction, and a complete definition of work would have to include this process. Work, therefore, is individually and socially constructed.

Work, for Hall, covers a broader range of activities than described above.

Housework is considered work, as is hustling (e.g., prostitution) or counterculture work (e.g., working in a kibbutz or as a Hare Krishna). Work can also be studied in horizontal (really the study of occupations) or vertical (work mobility, job change, etc.) dimensions. It is, however, the operation of work in an organizational context that, according to Hall, determines its nature. Thus, Hall presents a sociological perspective to the nature and determinants of work.

Neff (1985), in contrast, defines work as "an instrumental activity carried out by human beings, the object of which is to preserve and maintain life, which is directed at a planned alteration of certain features of man's environment" (p. 78). For Neff, work is a human activity that is performed to produce the means of subsistence and thereby maintain life, and that this occurs by man altering his environment. Work, therefore, is fundamentally a biological phenomenon that evolves in a social construct. Neff identifies his perspective as being consistent with a psychoanalytical approach to the understanding of work behavior. Feldman's research (1980) reflects a similar orientation, but now applied to the work history of the cancer patient.

Most psychological contributions have been in the area of the psychology of occupations, rather than the psychology of work. An occupation is a label attached to a social role or, to paraphrase Roe (1956, p. 3), "an occupation is whatever someone spends most of their time doing and thinking about." Psychologists' interest in occupations evolved out of studies of individual differences, the development of psychometric testing and evaluation, and the application of such tests to the study of vocational development. Studies of vocational development are particularly relevant for characterizing the long-term consequences of childhood cancer.

The above sample the economic, sociological, and psychological approaches to the definition of work (Tausky 1984). They illustrate the diversity of approaches and were not meant to be comprehensive. The definition of work proposed for this book might best be described as an ecological one, where work was considered only one component of a system of activities (see Moos [1986] for an extensive discussion of this approach). Judging the utility of a person's activities, such as a person with cancer, would have to involve all the activities the person engaged in, not just work-related activities. The distribution or redistribution of these activities and the social significance of these activities can be viewed from several perspectives. What has to be realized is that job discrimination is a product of a particular economic view (the market model), but that viable alternatives exist which would not make job discrimination a natural, unavoidable event.

WORK TRANSITIONS

The work history of an individual is marked by two major transition processes (Table 1.1): work establishment and work termination. Work establishment overlaps with a broad range of issues including occupational choice, vocational development, and occupational competence. It deals with the process whereby the nonworking child becomes the working adult. Work termination may be voluntary, involuntary, or involve self-imposed limitations. It may reflect a discriminatory event or the presence of a disability. It can lead to the assumption of a new role (a new job, unemployment, or retirement), or changes in a current job (work assignment, hours, etc.).

Work establishment, although described above as referring to a broad range of issues, is also used in a more narrow sense to refer to that period for the young (ages 25–35) during which the rate of job changing decreases (Freeman 1969). Or, stated differently, the probability of a person changing a job decreases as the duration of staying in a particular job increases. If this process leads to positions of greater prestige, then the person may be described as establishing a "career" (Wilensky 1961). While most workers do not have careers, in the sense described, most will go through the process of establishing a job.

Super, starting in 1951, has studied the career development of 300 14-year-old boys (Super 1985). Concurrently, he developed and tested a theory of vocational development. His theory states that vocational development is a lifelong process that starts somewhere in middle childhood. The individual is believed to pass through a series of stages defined as growth, exploration, establishment, maintenance, and decline. Not all of us follow this sequence of events, nor do we all progress at the same rate. Thus, some may have stable careers, some conventional, some unstable, and some multiple-trial careers. The key idea in Super's theory is that a person makes occupational choices that are consistent with his or her self-concept. What develops over time and with occupational experience is the person's self-concept. Occupational competence develops as the competence of the self develops.

Ginzberg, consistent with his interest in human resources, has also developed a theory of occupational choice (Ginzberg, et al. 1951). He, like Super, considers vocational development to be a process that starts in late childhood (ages 10–12) and continues into the twenties. What is unique about Ginzberg's theory is that he assumes that passage through the series of stages that mark occupational development produces irreversible decisions. Thus, early career decisions tend to reduce the degrees of freedom of later decision making. He also states that occupational decision making goes through stages: from fantasy (ages 10–12), to tentative (ages 12–17), to realistic (late adolescence to young adulthood). Factors both external and within the individual combine with these processes to produce an occupational outcome.

Anne Roe (1953,1956) has developed a theory of occupational interests based on in-depth studies of the personalities of working adults. She, unlike

Super and Ginzberg, is interested in early child-parent relationships and, like the psychoanalysts, believes that early parent and child interactions determine later personality and occupational choices. Unlike the analysts, she does not relate various periods of psychosexual development to the development of occupational identity, so that she cannot be considered to be taking a classical psychoanalytical perspective. Warm child-parent relationships, according to her theory, would lead the child to select a person-orientated occupation, while a cold rejecting family atmosphere would lead to nonperson-directed occupations (e.g., engineering).

One of the problems of applying what is known concerning occupational development to the cancer patient, particularly the childhood cancer survivor, is that the field itself is not that well developed. Roe (1964, pp. 211–12) reviewed the field in 1964, and her conclusions remain relevant today. She states that while there is some relationship between personality and occupation it is not a universal one. Personality is only one of several factors that contribute to occupational decisions. There is only sparse evidence relating early experience with latter occupational choices, although she would argue that appropriate studies have not been done. The occupational life history is never dependent upon one choice alone; many choices are involved.

These three theories just sample the available literature. What they have done is to provide a sketch of the options for putting together an approach to occupational development. Applying what is known to the study of the impact of cancer on occupational development requires that some estimates be available to determine if the level of occupational achievement for the individual with cancer deviates from what would have been expected. One way to assess a person's occupational achievements, without judging the social significance of the occupation, is to evaluate the competence with which individuals perform their jobs.

Occupational competence is a central conceptual issue in this book. It will play a major role in the research to be proposed, which will involve a shift from studies that try to prove that the cancer patient has been a victim of job discrimination to demonstrating that the cancer patient is work-able (that is, occupationally competent). Studies of job discrimination are analogous to studies of pathology; they attempt to identify the defect in a system that leads to a dysfunction. In contrast, studies of occupational competencies represent an effort to determine what leads to positive, effective functioning.

The concept of competence can be said to have originated with the development of the community mental health movement which started in the 1960s (Wine 1981). The community mental health movement has been described as a revolution in how psychological helping services are delivered (Levine & Levine 1970). It also greatly increased the need of social psychologists to understand how individuals respond to environmental demands; literally, how the individual copes with his environment. The characteristic of competence which permits this is its emphasis on evaluating the *effectiveness* with which an individual interacts with his or her environment, in which both the impact of the individual on the environment and environment on the individual are considered. Thus, competence has to be seen as a transactional variable. Competence is usually measured, in the psychological literature at least, in terms of overt behaviors, coping skills, and problem-solving abilities. It, however, has been defined in a variety of ways: as an intra-individual trait or disposition (Doll 1953), a motivational construct (White 1959), in terms of a list of accomplishments (Zigler & Phillips 1961), as specific overt behavioral coping skills (Hamburg & Adams 1967), or as a cognitive capacity (Goldfried & D'Zurilla 1969).

One of the attractive features of a competency model is that it also represents a shift in values. A human being is conceived of as growing, changing and learning as the person continuously interacts with his environment. In contrast, in the defect model efforts are made to identify sources of pathology or dysfunction and correct these problems. Defect interventions are not seen as contributing to the expression of human potential so much as removing obstacles to their expression (a passive role).

When applied to occupational issues, competence would also expect to reflect effectiveness, but now the effectiveness of job-related behaviors, coping skills, or problem-solving abilities. Occupational competence can be viewed as an end, as a reflection of a certain level of occupational activity (as the stage of a career), or as a process that can be disrupted. A particularly relevant example is the role that negative ideation plays in undermining social competence. It is relevant because it is the kind of event that would be expected to happen to a cancer patient who is considering continuing to work, changing a job, or asking for a raise. Negative ideation occurs when an individual reduces his or her self-esteem regarding some personal characteristic. An example would be if a person were to avoid a particular operation, convinced that he or she could not withstand the procedure (Kendall, et al. 1979). Expectancies, personal predictions about what will happen in a particular situation, also can impair social competency. An example of cognitive processes that facilitate social competence is problem-solving activities (Meichenbaum, et al. 1981). All-in-all there are a variety of ways in which an individual can think about him- or herself, contributing to or disrupting social (or occupational) competence. Unfortunately, these issues are rarely addressed in studies of job discrimination of the cancer patient primarily because there are few examples of the kind of prospective studies of the work history of the cancer patient required to generate the appropriate kind of data.

Performance appraisal is limited to an evaluation of a specific job or activity, while occupational competency reflects a more global evaluation of the work history of a person. Performance appraisal is an integral part of the work establishment and termination process. Three factors combine to determine its outcome: characteristics of the appraisee, the appraiser, and the context or environment where the appraisal is occurring (the work site). The appraisal context is best understood as contributing to ongoing processes in the appraisee and appraiser, and will not be discussed separately. The complexity of the appraisal process will illustrate the many ways by which it can lead to a discriminatory experience.

One of the determinants of the outcome of the appraisal process is how the person presents him- or herself. Schlenker (1980) refers to this as "impression management," or self-presentation. According to him, the way you present yourself when applying for a job, for example, is determined by automatic modes of behavior (which are well-learned behavioral scripts) or self-conscious types of behavior (as occur when a person acts deliberately to produce a particular outcome). The automatic modes of behavior reflect a person's "presence" ("he has appearance of an executive"), while the self-conscious types of behavior reflect persons controlling their behavior to produce particular outcomes (such as their dress, mannerisms, etc.). How having cancer impacts on either aspect of self-presentation is not known but it seems obvious that it would impact somehow.

The appraisal process itself is complex (Ilgen & Feldman 1983). Its function is to categorize stimuli and events that are then used in the judgment about people. Certain characteristics of an individual are appraised automatically or unconsciously (e.g., race, sex, or height); others are appraised by direct controlled attention. Automatic attentional processes exist to promote a "cognitive economy." The fact that attention occurs without volitional control means that irrelevant information about employees will be obtained despite the intentions of the appraiser. Direct controlled attention is also influenced by unintended and uncontrolled factors. The relevance of these processes for the performance appraisal of the cancer patient, or any patient with a chronic illness, seems obvious.

Categorization, which is the essential output in the appraisal process, also contributes to a cognitive economy—primarily by reducing the amount of information that must be processed and stored about an individual (Behling, et al. 1980). Automatic and controlled attentional components both contribute to the categorization process. Both must be developed by observation and learning (Rosch, et al. 1976). With time and repetition prototypical representations of the category develop and are used to evaluate characteristics of any individual. Thus, the experiences of the appraiser will be a major determinant of his assessment of the work-ableness of the cancer patient.

Figure 1.1 (Steers & Mowday 1981) illustrates a model of the elements that are involved in an employee's decision to change jobs. Changing jobs, however, is just one of several decisions that can lead to work termination.

Figure 1.1
A Simplified Model of Voluntary Turnover

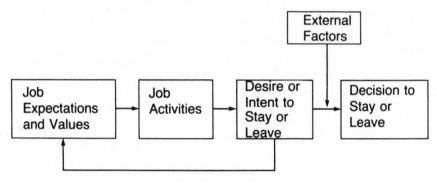

Modified from Figure 2, Steers and Mowday, *Research in Organizational Behavior*, 3, 1981, p. 242.

It will be used to illustrate the termination process. Every employee has certain expectations or values they associate with their job. These activities can determine the job activities of an employee, which are then expressed as desires or intentions by the person to stay or leave the job. The desires or intentions of the person are then reflected in the person's behavior. External factors, such as marital problems or having cancer, can influence the employee's desire and intent to stay or leave a job. The impact of external factors on the job intentions of the employee can lead to a search for alternatives: alternative job opportunities, alternative work arrangements, alternative work schedules, and so on.

Whether or not a person will actually change jobs will be critically dependent on the job market. If the market provides alternative opportunities, then this affects the person's expectations about the job and also his or her ultimate decision to stay or leave a job. Thus, perceived ease of movement between jobs is directly related to the desirability to move and ultimately the probability of a change in jobs.

Since having cancer ordinarily doesn't enhance one's marketability, this is not a major inducement for job change. Instead it may have the opposite effect—it may make the patient stay at a job for which he or she may be overqualified, not seek promotions, or simply not want to jeopardize his or her health insurance. It is at the level of job termination that the expression of self-imposed limitations is clearest (Barofsky 1982).

So far in this section we have discussed occupational development, occupational competence, performance appraisal, and job turnover. While these topics are not all that are relevant to the work transition process, they do illustrate the potential for analysis of the work history of the cancer patient. What is clear is that there are many issues that can be (but have not been as yet) formally addressed. Only after occupational development, occupational competence, and related topics have been studied, will it be possible to decide definitively if the cancer patient is a victim of job discrimination.

MODELS OF EMPLOYMENT DISCRIMINATION

Just as was found for work, there are economic and social-psychological definitions of employment discrimination. A clear, operational definition of employment discrimination is critical for both estimating its magnitude and basing policy initiatives. Most of what has been learned concerning economic models of employment discrimination is based on studies of discrimination against women or various racial groups (more recently the aged have been included in discrimination studies). The lack of economic studies of employment discrimination of persons with a particular disease reflects the small proportion of the population that may have the disease, and the political significance of such groups. Disease-related employment discrimination, however, should be accountable by the same economic and social psychological principles.

Webb (1891) argued that the reason why women are paid lower wages than men is because of the inelasticity of the female labor supply, or preferences or prejudices of employers. Both of these views reflect a market approach to discrimination. Women are paid less because they don't offer an employer much flexibility in terms of occupational preparation, ability to relocate, and capacity to stay employed at a particular job for an extended period. Each of these are characteristics of a labor supply that is less capable, less elastic than the demands of an employer may require.

Gary Becker (1957) developed a general theory of employment discrimination in a market economy based on an employer's "taste for discrimination." According to Becker, employers discriminate because they dislike having contact with members of one group, as opposed to another. The extent of their dislike can be measured by the employer's willingness to lose income so as to avoid contact with a particular group of people. Contact between the employer and the undesired group is dependent on the size of the group, the group's economic significance, and the duration and level of the contact. Sometimes the employer's preferences lead to wage discrimination, and sometimes to segregation.

While a cancer patient may be work-able, he still may be limited in terms of the jobs he can take (the inelasticity of the labor force). His employer may also want to segregate himself from the cancer patient since he symbolizes death and disability. Thus, the economic explanations offered to account for discrimination of women and minorities seem quite relevant to the cancer patient.

Gunnar Myrdal, in his classic *An American Dilemma* (1944), presents a model of discrimination based on the notion of "cumulative causation," or a vicious circle. Racial discrimination exists in the United States because of three factors, each of which feeds into the others summing to create the conditions for more discrimination. These factors are the presence of prejudices of whites against blacks; the economic status of blacks; and blacks' intelligence, ambitions, health, education, morals, or manners. Thus, whites look at the economic status and personal characteristics of blacks and feel justified in their prejudices and personal preferences, which then increases the probability that the employer will engage in discriminatory behavior again.

These two economic models of employment discrimination are important not only because they provide different explanations of why employment discrimination may occur but also because they provide the basis for designing preventive intervention programs. The market model assumes that economic characteristics alone, in a direct cause and effect manner, account for discriminatory behavior, while Myrdal's model requires a dynamic analysis that involves both economic and noneconomic factors. Intervention programs reflecting the market model would state that the economic issues raised by employing a cancer patient would have to be faced and resolved to prevent discriminatory employment practices, while the dynamic analysis of Myrdal would require studies of the pattern of cumulative causation so as to break the vicious circle that perpetuates the discriminatory behavior of employers. Neither of these two approaches has been formally tested, although they might have been if the initial phase of the RFP sponsored by the National Cancer Institute in 1973 had been successfully completed.

The method usually used to estimate the incidence of job discrimination objectively is an "actuarial" approach. This method has been successfully used to demonstrate the presence of race or sex discrimination. For example, approximately 15 percent of the U.S. population are minority group members. If a particular employer employs significantly fewer than 15 percent minority members then he may be considered to be discriminating. An actuarial approach to proving job discrimination against cancer patients, however, seems inappropriate. First, the cancer incidence rate for workers is quite low. Pell, et al. (1978), for example, estimated that the yearly cancer incidence rate for Dupont employees was only 2.2 percent, and the proportion of those who were work-able and could probably be discriminated against would be even lower. Such a low incidence rate increases the chances of errors of measurement and makes an actuarial approach to job discrimination of the cancer patient impractical.

One of the difficulties in studying employment discrimination is that it may involve several levels of analysis. Thus, discrimination may be characteristic of the beliefs of individuals, how organizations operate, or how a social system operates. Interestingly, it is probably easiest to change how a social system operates since legislative initiatives usually have "institutionalized" the discriminatory practices of the society. The classic example of this is the apartheid system of South Africa.

Figure 1.2
The Lack-of-Fit Model of Job Discrimination

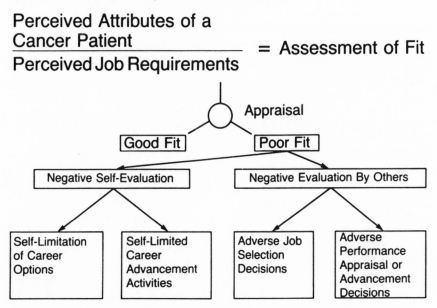

Adaptation of Figure 1, Heilman, *Research in Organizational Behavior, 5,* 1983, p. 281.

There are many opportunities for discriminatory acts to occur to the cancer patient and this is particularly evident at the organizational level of analysis. When they occur in the work environment they are harder to document and modify, although the sensitization of organizational practices and procedures to problems presented by the work-able cancer patient is a reasonable policy objective.

Much can be understood about the role of organizational factors in discriminatory events by an extension of the worker-to-job "fit" hypothesis to the cancer patient. This hypothesis, sometimes referred to as a "congruence" hypothesis, states that the objective characteristics of a worker's job and the values, needs, and social characteristics that the worker brings to the job have to match if the worker is to be satisfied with his or her job (Locke 1976; Mortimer 1979).

Heilman (1983) has extended the congruence hypothesis, stated as the "lack of fit" model, in an effort to understand sex bias in the work setting, and her notions will be extended further to understand the discriminatory experience of the cancer patient (Figure 1.2). She points out that two characteristics of organizational behavior, sex stereotyping and sex typing of jobs, are major determinants of sex bias. The same may be true for the cancer patient.

A stereotype is a generalization that is made about a group that is applied to individuals. The generalization that all cancer patients die prematurely, have marked physical limitations, receive extended treatment and generate large medical costs is a classic example of a stereotype. The existence of such a stereotype puts the work–able cancer patient on the defensive; he or she has to prove their capacity to work under conditions that others would not.

To what extent is the work-ableness of a cancer patient a function of a stereotype or real differences between cancer and noncancer patients? When a similar question is asked about differences between the sexes, then the answer is found to be very dependent on the assessment method. Thus, verbal reports (which are highly susceptible to influences from stereotypes and other expectancies) are found to reveal larger differences between the sexes than direct observation (Maccoby & Jacklin 1974). A similar dependence on the assessment method should be found for the cancer patient. A cancer patient, believing the stereotype about his/her work-ableness, may actually dismiss discriminatory experiences as a normal part of the working environment, and underreport work discrimination events. Alternatively, the cancer patients may overreport their work-related needs, the problem of questionnaire reactivity. These methodological issues confound estimates of magnitude of employment discrimination of the cancer patient, but also reflect the dynamics operating in an organization.

Just as there is sex typing of jobs, so too there is "cancer typing" of jobs. A classic example of this is the, until recently, nearly complete refusal of the armed forces to permit cancer patients to enlist or remain in the services. Somehow the armed forces had determined that the requirements of being a soldier excluded someone who has or had cancer. They had argued that the label "cancer" was irreversible, and that a childhood or adult cancer survivor could never be considered to be totally combat ready. Alternatively, the armed services may have considered the psychological burden of having had cancer to impair the person's capacity to withstand the psychological burden of combat. Independent of the logic, it appears that the armed services judged that the perceived attributes of all cancer patients and the perceived job requirements of a soldier did not match, illustrating the "lack of fit" hypothesis.

The potential for cancer stereotyping and cancer typing of jobs makes the lack-of-fit model an appropriate approach to the measurement of job discrimination. Only the Fobair, et al. study (Chapter 6, this volume) is known to have directly applied this model to the cancer patient.

STUDIES OF THE WORK HISTORY OF THE CANCER PATIENT

The next chapters deal with the work and insurance experiences of the cancer patient. The results of these studies will be reviewed in Chapter 8

Table 1.2
Sample Requirements of the Work-Able Project

Contractor	Required Sample		SMSAs
	Employers	Patients	
A	225	150	Pittsburgh, Akron, San Francisco
B	300	150	Boston, Atlanta, New Orleans
C	225	150	Richmond, Denver, Minneapolis/St. Paul
D	204	150	New York City, St. Louis, Houston
E	180	150	Baltimore, Seattle, Miami
	1134	750	

Source: L. D. Burke and G. E. Metter, Review of the Work-able Contract, Division of Resources, Centers and Community Activities, National Cancer Institute, 1980.

(Barofsky, this volume). What will be discussed in some detail is the outcome of the NCI–sponsored Work-able Project, a project the scope and intent of which remains the most ambitious effort, to date, to effect the discriminatory experience of cancer patients (Bloom, et al. 1976; Counts, et al. 1976; Reynolds 1977; Smith, et al. 1977; Wilson, et al. 1976). Its universally acknowledged failure provides a model of what needs to be attended to for the successful implementation of a project of this sort (Burke & Metter, 1980). It also provides an opportunity to bring into focus the fact that the discriminatory experience of the cancer patient may require a different analytical approach than was used to demonstrate discrimination in minority groups, women, and so on.

The plan of the study was to interview both employers and employees. The surveys were conducted in 15 Standard Metropolitan Statistical Areas (SMSAs) across the United States. The SMSAs were chosen to produce a broad distribution of firms that would include: a variety of types of industries (mining, manufacturing, services, etc.), major labor markets (New York, Pittsburgh, Atlanta, etc.), and geographic dispersion. The study was to interview 750 patients and 1134 employers (Table 1.2).

The employers survey was to be conducted among a stratified cluster sample of business firms in each SMSA. The survey dealt with the employer's attitudes, policies, and practices relative to the employment of patients with a history of cancer. Eight types of employers (agriculture, construction, manufacturing, transportation, retail trade, etc.) and four sizes

Table 1.3
Sample Selection and Interview Completion Rates for Employer Survey by Contractor

CONTRACTOR

Number of Employers in:

	A	B	C	D	E
Initial Sample Selected:	376	552	Not given	299	Not given
Exclusions Initial Sample:	75	56	(about 20%)	76	Not given
Interviews Not Completed	77	265	High	34	Not given
Completed Interviews	223	231	286	189	265
Percent Completed	74%	47%	?	>63%, <85%	?

Source: Burke and Metter, 1980.

of employers (100–249, 250–499, 500–999, 1000 or more) made up a 32-cell sampling frame. A Dun and Bradstreet listing was used to select up to nine firms per cell randomly for a total of 228 firms per SMSA (4320 total firms selected). Oversampling (Table 1.2) was designed to compensate for the potential refusal of employers to participate in the survey.

The patient survey was to be a one time telephone survey of 750 (50 per SMSA) persons with a history of cancer. The survey covered the patients' work history following their therapy. The sample was limited to workable persons who had invasive cancer, were diagnosed one to three years prior, and resided in the area of the tumor registry used to identify the sample. The sample was stratified on the basis of age (20–29, 30–44, 45–59), sex, and condition of health (disease-free, or other).

Five consulting firms were selected to implement the contract. Table 1.3 summarizes the sample selection and interview completion rate for the

Table 1.4
Sample Selection and Interview Completion Rate for Patient Survey by Contractor

CONTRACTOR

Number of Patients in:

	A	B	C	D	E
Initial Sample Selected	396	Not given	600 (?)	641	Not given
Physician Permission Granted	379	Not given	192	370	1051
Interviews Not Given	243	Not given	97(?)	275	Not given
Interviews Consented To	136	154	95(?)	95	Not given
Completed Interviews	123	140	92	95	101
Percent Completed	31%	?	15%(?)	15%	?

Source: Burke and Metter, 1980.

employer survey as available in the contractor's final reports. What is immediately obvious is that each contractor was not as systematic in his or her efforts to summarize activities as the others, precluding any hope of pooling the available data. The same can be said for the patient survey (Table 1.4). Contractors also differed in the types of statistical analyses that were performed, also precluding pooling efforts.

The contractors ran into major accrual problems for both surveys. This was partially due to the fact that the Dun and Bradstreet listing was not up-to-date so that a proportion of the firms listed were out of business and should have not been included in the original sample (Burke & Metter, 1980). This included as much as 10–20 percent of the initial sample. However, of those employers eligible to be interviewed 26 percent for one contractor and 53 percent for another refused to participate (Table 1.2). Some contractors did not provide the information required to report the nonresponse rate (Table 1.2). Thus, there was a profound accrual bias in the sample even for those contractors that reported the data. It is, of course, possible that those firms that were not interviewed engaged in discriminatory practices, so that the inference drawn by several of the contractors that there was minimal discrimination seems moot, or at best a minimal figure.

The contractors ran into similar accrual problems for the patient survey, particularly as regards obtaining permission from the tumor registries to use their records for selection of the sample and physicians to contact their patients. In addition, even if permission was given, the interview completion rate was quite low, ranging form 10 to 48 percent. When given, the reasons for noncompletion included refusals or failure to respond to requests for interview, and inability to locate individuals. What was particularly vexing was the fact that a large proportion of the patients interviewed had not sought employment since their cancer, so that they should not have been incorporated into the study sample to begin with.

One contractor's data (Contractor A) was more complete than others and will, therefore, be used to summarize the results of the study. First, only 123 of the initial 396 patients were successfully interviewed. Of the remaining patients, however, only 23 sought employment following their treatment for cancer, and of these six (23%) reported discriminatory events associated with their job. Eighteen percent of the employer sample felt that they would not hire a work-able cancer patient. Physician's working for firms uniformly requested more physical evaluation of cancer patients than other patients.

Several "lessons" can be learned from the Work-able Project. First, it seemed clear that this project, coming at the time that the Cancer Rehabilitation Program was starting, was premature and overly ambitious. It proceeded in a political climate which assumed, as was found useful for minority discrimination studies, that retrospective self-reports would be sufficient to demonstrate the existence of discrimination. Second, it assumed that there would be no problems for an "outside" contractor to gain access to the cancer care system, if it were clear that they were representing the National Cancer Institute. This was clearly not the case. Third, it was evident that the cooperation between the funding agency and contractee is critical to the outcome no matter how well designed the study. This effort might have been significantly more successful if initially a series of smaller, more focused studies had been done to provide the investigators with a sense of the research problems that a large study would create. The study also lacked a visible epidemiological input, something which would still be an issue today. Thus, the power of the inferences possible from estimates of the magnitude of job discrimination of the cancer patient remain limited

Table 1.5
Summary of Employment Discrimination Studies*

Author(s)	N	Discrimination Measure
Feldman (1976)	130	22% of sample reports at least one job rejection due to cancer.
Counts etal (1976)	26	23% of sample reports discriminatory experience.
Smith etal (1977)	95	13.7% of sample report at least one job rejection due to cancer.
Forster, etal (1979)	60	40% of sample reports job discrimination.
Fobair, etal (1986)	403	42%(?) of sample reports job related problems

* Partial list

Source: Compiled by author.

(Table 1.5) with most studies consisting of small convenience samples that use retrospective surveys and lack independent confirmation of the discriminatory experience. More recent studies have included control groups and have helped place the data on job discrimination of the cancer patient on a firmer empirical foundation.

SUMMARY

Clearly, the work history of the cancer patient is a subject that is worth studying in its own right. It provides a model of how external events, the occurrence and treatment of a disease, impacts the work process. It, therefore, is a legitimate component of the psychology and sociology of work. Since the cancer patient is a member of the labor force, the study of the impact of cancer and other chronic diseases on the labor market is a legitimate activity for economic study. However, the reason why the job discriminatory experiences of the cancer patient should be studied is not just because it is academically interesting but because of the profound human consequences of the experience. Not only does it reflect a diminished quality of life, it also reflects the fact that a person is falling victim to an imperfect social system, a system that requires active correction if it is to succeed in achieving its stated goals. To state that an injustice is being perpetrated against the cancer patient who has a discriminatory experience does not mean that he or she is unique or singled out for this experience. There may be many examples of such injustices, some even more unfair than what the cancer patient experiences, but all require rectification.

One of the ways to approach the design of interventions for an action program is to study the conditions under which cancer, and not the person's qualifications for the job, becomes a determinant of their work status. This chapter has reviewed a number of such variables that may be worth studying.

REFERENCES

Barofsky, I. Job discrimination: A measure of the social death of the cancer patient. In *Proceedings of the western states conference on cancer rehabilitation*. Palo Alto, CA: Bull, 1982.

Becker, G. S. *The economics of discrimination*. Chicago: University of Chicago, 1957.

Behling, V. W., Gifford, W. E., & Tolliver, J. M. Effects of grouping information on decision making under risk. *Decision Sciences*, 1980, *11*, 272–283.

Bergermaier, R., Borg, I., & Champoux, J. E. Structural relationships among facets of work, nonwork and general well-being. *Work and Occupation*, 1984, *11*, 163–181.

Bloom, M. V., Rosenberg, B., & Novallis, C. N. *Modification of employer's attitudes toward the employment of work-able cancer patients*. Final Report. 2 Vols. Silver Spring, MD: Applied Management Sciences, 1976.

Burke, L. D., & Metter, G. E. Review of the work-able contract. Division of Resources, Centers and Community Activities, National Cancer Institute, 1980.

Campbell, A. *The sense of well-being in America: Recent patterns and trends*. New York: McGraw-Hill, 1981.

Counts, S., Rodov, M. H., & Wilson, M. T. *Attitudes of employers and cancer patients toward patients' work ability: Two surveys and an action plan*. 2 Vols. Prepared for the National Cancer Institute. Pittsburgh, PA: American Institutes for Research, Center for Health Systems Studies, 1976.

Doll, E. A. *Measurement of social competence*. Minneapolis, MI: Educational Test Bureau, 1953.

Feldman, F. L. *Work and cancer health histories: Work expectations and experiences of youth with cancer histories (ages 13–23)*. Oakland: California Division, American Cancer Society, 1980.

Freeman, M. *The process of work establishment*. New York: Columbia, 1969.

Ginzberg, E. *The human economy*. New York: McGraw-Hill, 1976.

Ginzberg, E., Ginsburg, S. W., Axelrad, S., & Herma, J. L. *Occupational choice: An approach to a general theory*. New York: Columbia, 1951.

Goldfried, M. R., & D'Zurilla, T. J. A behavioral-analytic model for assessing competence. In C. D. Spielberger (Ed.), *Current topics in clinical and community psychology*. New York: Academic, 1969.

Hall, R.H.H. *Dimensions of work*. Beverly Hills, CA: Sage, 1986.

Hamburg, D. A., & Adams, J. E. A perspective on coping behavior. *Archives of General Psychiatry*, 1967, *17*, 277–284.

Heilman, M. E. Sex bias in work settings: The lack of fit model. *Research in Organizational Behavior*, 1983, *5*, 269–298.

Ilgen, D. R., & Feldman, J. M. Performance appraisal: A process focus. *Research in Organizational Behavior*, 1983, *5*, 141–197.

Kendall, P., Williams L., Pechacek, T., Graham, L., Shisslak, C., & Herzoff, N. Cognitive-behavioral and patient education in catheterization procedures. *Journal of Consulting and Clinical Psychology*, 1979, *47*, 49–58.

Levine, M., & Levine, A. *A social history of helping services: Clinic, court, school and community.* New York: Appleton-Century-Crofts, 1970.

Locke, E. A. The nature and causes of job satisfaction. In M. D. Dunnette (Ed.), *Handbook of Industrial and Organizational Psychology.* Chicago: Rand McNally, 1976.

Maccoby, E. E., & Jacklin, C. N. *The psychology of sex differences.* Stanford, CA: Stanford University, 1974.

McKenna, R. J. Analysis of case histories: Re-employment problems of the recovered cancer patient. A report by the Ad Hoc Subcommittee on Employability of the Recovered Cancer Patient. San Francisco: California Division, American Cancer Society, Inc., 1973.

Meichenbaum, D., Butler, L., & Gruson, L. Toward a conceptual model of social competence. In J. D. Wine & M. D. Smye (Eds.), *Social competence.* New York: Guilford, 1981.

Moos, R. H. Work as a human context. In M. S. Paak & R. Peroff (Ed.), *Psychology and work: Productivity, change, and employment.* Washington, DC: American Psychological Association, 1986.

Mortimer, J. T. *Changing attitudes toward work.* Scarsdale, NY: Work in America Institute, 1979.

Myrdal, G. *An American dilemma: The Negro problem and modern democracy.* 2 Vols. New York: Harper, 1944.

National Cancer Rehabilitation Planning Conference. Chairman's Report: Rehabilitation Planning Report. June 19, 1973.

Neff, W. S. *Work and human behavior.* 3rd ed. New York: Aldine, 1985.

Pell, S., O'Berg, M. T., & Karrh, B. W. Cancer epidemiologic surveillance in the Du Pont company. *Journal of Occupational Medicine*, 1978, *20*, 725–740.

Request for proposal (RFP). *Modification of employer's attitude toward the employment of work-able cancer patients.* Division of Cancer Control and Rehabilitation, National Cancer Institute, December 20, 1973.

Reynolds, J. *The employability of work-able cancer patients. Executive summary. Findings, conclusions, and recommendations: Survey of employers and patients in New York, St. Louis, and Houston.* No. 2. Prepared for the National Cancer Institute. University Research Corporation, 1977.

Roe, A. *The making of a scientist.* New York: Dodd, Mead, 1953.

Roe, A. Personality structure and occupational behavior. In H. Borow (Ed.), *Man in a world of work.* Boston: Houghton Mifflin, 1964.

Roe, A. *The psychology of occupations.* New York: Wiley, 1956.

Rosch, E. Human categorization. In N. Warren (Ed.), *Studies in cross-cultural psychology.* Vol. 1. New York: Academic, 1977.

Smith, L., Jr., Seboda, B. L., Blinzley, R. J., & Wood, D. *Employment practices and the work-able cancer patient. Final report.* 2 Vols. Prepared for the National Cancer Institute. Westinghouse Health Systems, 1977.

Steers, R. M., & Mowday, R. T. Employee turnover and post-decision accommodation processes. *Research in Organizational Behavior,* 1981, *3,* 235–281.

Super, D. E. Coming of age in Middletown: Careers in the making. *American Psychologist,* 1985, *40,* 405–414.

Tausky, C. *Work and society: An introduction to industrial sociology.* Itasca, IL: Peacock, 1984.

Webb, S. The alleged differences in the wages paid to men and women for similar work. *Economics Journal,* 1891, *1,* 635–662.

White, R. Motivation reconsidered: The concept of competence. *Psychological Review,* 1959, *66,* 297–333.

Wilensky, H. L. Orderly careers and social participation: The impact of work history on social integration in the middle mass. *American Sociological Review,* 1961, *26,* 523–563.

Wilson, T. R., Richards, J. A., & Bercini, D. H. *A study of the employment of work-able cancer patients: Survey of employer attitudes and practices.* Final Report. Prepared for the National Cancer Institute. Human Resources Research Organization, 1976.

Wine, J. D. From defect to competence models. In J. D. Wine & M. D. Smye (Eds.), *Social Competence.* New York: Guilford, 1981.

Zigler, E., & Phillips, L. Social competence and outcome in psychiatric disorder. *Journal of Abnormal and Social Psychology,* 1961, *63,* 264–271.

2

Inquiries into Work Experiences of Recovered Cancer Patients: The California Experience

Frances Lomas Feldman

When I returned to work, my desk had been moved away from all the others. I'd sat in the same spot in the center of the secretarial pool for twelve years. Now I was consigned to this new location, a pariah separated from the others by a bank of green steel files. My supervisor said I'd have quiet and privacy—that I knew I didn't need!

To guard the other students from the dangers of contamination, I arranged a special table to be brought in and put a bit away from the desks of the others in the classroom.

What could have caused such actions? They were provoked by cancer, reported by respondents in a trilogy of studies that sought to learn about the work experiences of individuals after they had been diagnosed as having cancer (Feldman 1976; 1978; 1980). In the first instance, the worker had undergone surgery to remove a malignant polyp from the throat. Not only did she feel well enough to resume a full working schedule, there were neither visible nor audible evidences of the diagnosis or treatment. In the second instance, the teacher described the return of 16-year-old Hugh to the classroom following a diagnosis of Hodgkin's disease. Both incidents, initially disclosed by the patient and then affirmed by co-workers or school personnel, reflect societal and personal perceptions of cancer that have deep roots in antiquity and continue to impact profoundly the quality of the cancer patient's life.

Without in any way comparing the etiology or symptomatology of any form of cancer to other chronic diseases, it nevertheless is noteworthy that panicky fear and revulsion, reminiscent of attitudes in evidence for centuries toward individuals with cancer, remains today. These attitudes persist despite extensive public information and education about origins of cancer and progress in its containment, control, and cure. For enhanced public sophistication about causes, course, and control of cancer has not eliminated tenacious vestigial beliefs that it is shameful, a contaminant, and, among other opinions rooted in folklore, doubtlessly a punishment visited on the victim for unidentifiable actions or thoughts that induce a pervasive sense of guilt in the patient. Such superstitious remnants from the past often blur with discomfort in the individual who does not have cancer but "can't act natural" in the presence of someone who today is faced with a seemingly life-threatening illness. One consequence of such attitudinal manifestations is exacerbation of the stress and distress inherent in the patient's struggle to cope with the diagnosis and treatment of the disease.

In a work-oriented society like ours that places a high premium on productive attachment of adults to the work force, what attitudes (with what effects) are encountered by persons who seek to enter or reenter the world of work following a diagnosis of cancer? Whether negative or positive, what is the significance of such attitudes for the well-being of the individual patient, for public policy, for public and professional education about cancer?

The content and the inferences offered in this chapter derive in large measure from three formal studies conducted by the author about work experiences of individuals following a diagnosis of cancer. It examines ways in which the original research design endeavored to elicit understanding of how and why the experiences took their course and the measures that were instituted in the subsequent studies to correct for weaknesses or gaps in the earlier study. The chapter also draws on subsequent structured and informal undertakings and experiences of the author and others that reinforce the learnings from the trilogy or illuminate further the work-related coping needs and patterns of individuals still attached to the work force following a bout with cancer.

WORK AND THE CANCER PATIENT

The life-threatening nature of cancer often evokes in the patient and others an almost overwhelming image of inexorably painful and deadly disease. The patient's attitudes about cancer may combine with attitudes of those around him or her to reinforce a sense of lack of control over the progress of the cancer and, by extension, over him- or herself and the quality of life. How will co-workers and others in the work setting react to this diminished self? With pity? With resentment or apprehension that the returning patient is a pariah, unable to perform requisite work tasks without undue reliance on co-workers? How will the patient be able to demonstrate continuing capability for managing his or her work, for controlling affairs and self, and demonstrate that he or she is an independent, adequately functioning individual? For the likelihood is that the individual has grown up incorporating certain societal expectations that equate economic and psychological independence with adequacy as an adult, that pair independence with working and earning, and that perceive working and earning as contingent on reasonably good (and continuing) health. A diagnosis of cancer in and of itself almost invariably is a profound source of stress; the emotional vulnerability of the cancer patient with a strong work ethic—and not infrequently, his or her economic vulnerability as well—is intensified if the individual perceives his or her work status to be in jeopardy.

Work properly refers to any activity in which an individual engages that produces something of value for other people (O'Toole 1974). This definition includes the varied tasks of the homemaker as well as the community volunteer. For purposes of this chapter, as in the Work and Cancer series, "work" refers to *paid* employment, wherever and whenever it is performed and regardless of its nature. When examined against this definition, the concept that human beings are not born with ability to work may strike some readers as heretical or, at the very least, immoral. *How* to work has been learned through events and circumstances within a complex matrix of sociocultural expectations, requirements, demands, strictures, and environmental and other conditions (Neff 1985). *Why* one should work is not an economic function alone: It also is a phenomenon driven by myriad social forces, often fueled by religious ideology as advocated by sixth century Benedictines (Bettenson 1947) or religious controversy centered around the Protestant Reformation (Weber 1930)—or even, as Tawney (1926) believed, the aspirations of a new and rising class of merchants.

The idea that work is a virtue came to America from Europe, nurtured at first by pioneer rigors of defense and survival. It has been reinforced by the personal traditions of hard work brought by immigrants from Asia as well as by particular conditions of life in the United States that have underscored its personal and national importance and given it a special quality. Wherever its roots and however nourished, conceptions of work have been glorified persistently in our culture: Work is intrinsically good. In a nation with a strong and abiding heritage of rugged individualism and independence of person and spirit, work has come to represent adequacy; it often is a moral and psychological index to one's value as a human being, a manifestation of worthiness and respectability—and if respect is merited from others, clearly *self*-respect also is in order. Hence, in work we see factors that affect our sense of our own value or self-esteem, identity, and dignity: ingredients essential for effective management or social functioning in our society (Feldman & Scherz 1968).

What is in work for the person with a diagnosis of cancer? What are the implications for the cancer patient who has incorporated a work-oriented value system fostered in a work-ethic environment that fails to accord the individual full or continuing membership? What is the significance for the young person whose developmental dependence–independence struggle occurs against a backdrop of treatment for pediatric cancer and whose planning for a future education or vocational choice is clouded by questions about survival? To a considerable degree the autonomy of the patient with cancer is lessened. Regardless of the cause of the cancer, its reality is equated with diminution of mastery over oneself, of control over one's own destiny. What is the consequence for the individual when this threat to autonomy is compounded by questions about continued attachment to the work force even though the cancer is in remission, if not cured, and the individual feels able to work?

Over a period of several years, a growing number of written and verbal complaints were brought to the attention of the California Division of the American Cancer Society by a complainant or an interested third party (a relative or friend, or the physician) protesting work discrimination attributed to a cancer diagnosis. These had been carefully assembled and clinically analyzed by Dr. Robert McKenna (1973), then chairman of the Division's ad hoc Committee on Employability Problems of the Recovered Cancer Patient. The poignant pattern of acute distress and depression that emerged prompted wonder in the Division about the magnitude of such discrimination as a social problem and about the nature of the Division's responsibility with respect to its alleviation. And out of this dual concern emerged the decision to sponsor the effort to seek data about the nature of work experiences of persons with cancer histories.

THE WORK AND CANCER HEALTH HISTORIES STUDIES

Aside from Dr. McKenna's report and occasional print and electronic news media dramatizations of appealing human interest accounts of individual experiences that connected cancer and work discrimination, there had been a paucity of systematic inquiry about any relationship between cancer and work prior to the trilogy. Two studies had been conducted about the post-cancer performance of individuals employed by the Metropolitan Life Insurance Company (Wheatley et al. 1974) and the American Telephone and Telegraph Company (Stone 1975). However, although they and the McKenna report contain useful clues to understanding the drive to work and the productivity of employed cancer patients, the McKenna compilation necessarily was confined to a self-selected population characterized by generally unconfirmed work problems, and the other two compared the wide spectrum of work experiences and performance of work-able cancer patients with those of other employees in their respective companies. None addressed the experiences of recovered cancer patients in the population at large.

What would be shown by a study of experiences of patients randomly drawn from a wider population of persons with a history of cancer? Does the reality of a cancer history affect work opportunities and experiences? If so, under what circumstances, in what ways, and with what implications for the individual as well as society? It was to obtain some insights into such questions that the trilogy of Work and Cancer studies was undertaken under the auspices of the California Division of the American Cancer Society.

Several conditions in particular governed the course of this research and merit prefatory comment. One is that even though incidents of alleged cancer-related discrimination in the world of work precipitated the Division's decision to support the research, there was clear understanding from the outset that the focus would be on work *experiences,* positive and negative. Another was financial constraint. The division had elected to make available a small year-end sum that had not been needed for its originally budgeted purposes: The resulting study was tailored to take into account the amount of skilled research interviewing time this sum could purchase in addition to essential supplies, postage, and report preparation.[1] In contrast to a rather precipitous decision to utilize the unexpectedly available funds for the first study, the next two had more adequate lead time for developing the research and funding plans.

Designing the Studies

The focus of the first study (WC) was on persons in white collar occupations and in the fields of nursing or teaching. This decision was motivated by a labor market that was relatively favorable to these occupations when the study was being planned: It seemed likely that experiences of a sample of patients from these groups might be conservatively predictive of experiences among occupational groups for whom employment opportunities might be less accessible, whether or not the persons had ever had cancer. The second study then was addressed to blue collar and service occupations (BC). The construction of samples in the youth study (YS) was not by occupation, although this element was included in data analysis.

Other than occupation, similar criteria guided construction of the patient samples in the adult studies. Holding a job at the time of the cancer diagnosis was regarded as pragmatic evidence that the individual was attached to the work force. The age range, 23 to 50 years at diagnosis, was utilized so that younger patients would have had some qualifying work experience and older patients under ordinary circumstances could anticipate a work life of at least 10 additional years. Susceptibility to job exclusion because of ageism—too young or too old—would thus be minimized. Three cancer site groups were over-represented, because of the frequency of their incidence and because of their relatively favorable survival rates: breast, head/neck, and rectum/colon. It was expected that some of the patients would offer visible evidence of surgical treatment.

Patients in the youth study were not screened by site, their only requisite being they were survivors of cancer diagnosed when they were in the age range of 13 to 23 years at diagnosis. This wide span of years was selected for two reasons: It would bridge the middle-school years, when vocational planning often begins, through college or to the point of entering a career; and it encompassed the several developmental stages, from the early adolescent years through the late or extended adolescent years, any or all of which stages would bear in their unique ways upon the coping behavior of the respondent. Because the interviews would occur from one to five years after diagnosis, it was expected that some respondents would still be in school, while others would be in or trying to enter the labor force.

From the start the study designers dealt with two congeries of issues. One included feasible and ethical processes for procuring the participation of individual patients. The other encompassed measures by which to corroborate, validate, or refute patients' perceptions of cancer-related work or school experiences that necessarily would be retrospective and shaped by emotions, distance in time, and other elements that influence memory. Comprehensive searches for relevant published and unpublished literature had failed to disclose useful guidelines pertinent to psychosocial research on work experiences of work-able patients with a cancer (or other) health history. Protocols had to be devised that would not render the data or findings susceptible to skepticism because of the absence of recourse to control or comparison groups. Furthermore, there was cognizance that responses might be affected by a climate redolent with heightened sensitivity among health professionals about protecting confidentiality and about medical malpractice threats, among employing establishments about affirmative action and fair employment practice issues and problems, and among various interests concerned with procuring truly informed consents from potential respondents.

Some of the questions and answers that were taken into account in fashioning the studies so that a reasonably accurate picture of cancer-related work experiences would emerge, are identified in the following paragraphs; the consequences and implications of their implementation are presented subsequently.

Patient Selection

The university-based research team benefited enormously form the existence and involvement of the centralized registry, the Cancer Surveillance Program (CSP), that had been established in 1970 as part of a comprehensive and interdisciplinary research project on cancer virus within the Comprehensive Cancer Center in the University of Southern California's Medical School. All hospitals in Los Angeles County—and those in adjacent counties that might have Los Angeles residents as patients—supplied demographic data to the Program gathered by the Program's own health professionals who regularly visited the 177 participating hospitals to collect, store, and protect these data. More than 20,000 malignancies were recorded each year. With the exception of several small hospitals that were known in advance to refuse to be involved in any research that called for contact with their patients or doctors, the computerized records were read to obtain a count of possible respondents from each hospital. A two-year time frame was used with the hope of obtaining at least 80 respondents for each of the two adult studies. To obtain at least 75 youth respondents, five years of computer records were read. The sheer size of this single county's geography and population as well as its diversity by reason of rural-urban distribution, agriculture and manufacturing, multi-ethnic and multi-cultural variations, and economic spread, suggested that the desired samples would be comparable in many respects to the study populations that might be drawn from the aggregate of several other states.

To the hospitals with potential patient-respondents (the computerized files had not reported surviving patients who met the study criteria in all the hospitals), a request was sent for authorization to compile a roster of patients and their physicians of record, and for permission to approach the doctors about obtaining the patients' participation in the respective study. When such authorization was received, a letter went to the physician explaining the purpose of the study and asking permission to contact the patient and for notation of any reservations the doctor might have about communication with the patient by the researchers. Only on receipt of this signed authorization was a letter dispatched to the patient to describe the study objectives and enclose, along with the stamped return envelope, an authorization-to-interview on which the potential respondent could note convenient times and means for arranging an interview appointment or asking for more information about the study. In the youth study, such letters were sent not just to all potential patient-respondents (regardless of age) but also to parents or guardians of minors. A second letter went to doctors, parents, or patients who had not answered the first; there was a telephone follow-up with nonresponding physicians, but not with patients or parents.

This time-consuming multi-step process was governed by considerations about principles for protecting confidentiality and assuring that consent was truly informed. But it also paid cautious attention to phrasing queries so that responses about work or school experiences would not be skewed in the direction of negative or positive experiences; and, in the instance of young people and their parents or guardians, there was cognizance that it was important not just to acknowledge parental legal rights in decision making about their children's participation, but also to accord the latter recognition as persons capable of speaking on their own behalf. The latter simple step turned out to have a special effect on the quality and direction of some of the subsequent research interviews, the young person's responsiveness clearly influenced by acceptance as a thinking person in his or her own right.

Validation of Responses

In the Metropolitan Life Insurance Company and the American Telephone and Telegraph Company studies it was possible to compare the work behavior and productivity of the employees with cancer histories and the work behavior and productivity of co-workers with other kinds of health histories. But such counterpart samples could not be constructed practically or validly in the Work and Cancer trilogy.

The studies aimed to obtain both qualitative and quantitative data that might shed light on the relationship between an individual's cancer history and work experiences. The patient's self-perception that he or she was able to work and still was attached to the work force was confirmed by the doctor's authorization to the research team to communicate with the patient. This view of the patient as work-able in many instances distinguished the WC and BC samples from those in other studies that included some consideration of the work experiences of cancer patients.

The critical perceptions of how the patient had fared in the world of work following the diagnosis were irrefutably the patients'. But how accurate would that perception be in view of the filtering system to which memory is subject over time and that more or less shapes the distillate? That the patient might *feel* he or she is a victim of unfairness or discrimination in the workplace because of the cancer certainly can be taken as fact; the extent to which that fact is rooted in objective reality, however, requires attestation.

What could comprise such testimony? This was a major concern is designing the WC research. In part to reconnoiter this question and in part to test the interview instruments, individual exploratory conferences were held with patients volunteered by their physicians and with (haphazardly) selected personnel managers and executives in several industrial and government organizations. In addition, invitations were sent by local units of the American Cancer Society to known patients, asking them to join the principal investigators in one of three meetings held for the purpose of refining instruments and protocols with their participation. Not only did the individuals and groups respond freely to the invitation critically to examine the inclusion, exclusion, language, and order to queries; they also addressed the question of validating employment information and work patterns of patient-respondents.

The original staffing plan had called for a labor-management specialist with high-level research interviewing experience and skills. It now was agreed that any documentary items a patient or employer might make available, such as letters or notifications of change in work status or assignment, would be scrutinized, but several additional measures would be followed. One was to interview a purposive sample (20 percent) of employing establishments represented in the patient sample. When an authorization had been supplied by the patient to contact the employer and such an approach would not threaten the employee's work status or relationships, interviews were conducted with several levels of personnel in order to note similar or different understandings and practices within the organization both with respect to the identified employee and in general. If the patient was uneasy about such contact, or the interviewer thought the patient vulnerable in some way, a different but similar organization was approached about its policies and practices with regard to hiring or retaining personnel with a cancer history. When possible, if a patient had reported questionable or unfavorable treatment in a particular work environment, that organization and a comparable one were included in the employer sample. To illustrate, if a patient authorized contact with a prior or current employer in a school district, another school district also was approached to ascertain similarities in relevant policies or variations in how they were implemented; when a tire manufacturing plant was named by a patient, a similar kind of manufacturing concern was visited. This interview phase yielded understanding of policies, practices, and attitudes that affected a given patient-respondent and cancer patients in general. It likewise offered a picture of similarities and/or differences in policy interpretations and in attitudes about cancer among various levels within a particular organization and, also, among two or more like organizations.

A second measure was designed to assess the validity of the specific patient-respondent's report of cancer-related work problems. Armed with 12 consents from patients that had been randomly pulled from among all the consents, the employment interviewer traced the employee-reported experiences with pre-cancer and post-cancer employers and, where possible, potential employers in the post-diagnosis period. The dyads were expected to yield some clues to the patients' work behavior patterns both before and after the illness and to add or deny credence to the reported occurrence of discrimination or other cancer-related work problems. The interview schedule allowed for structured and open-ended responses and was supplemented when possible with examination of such personnel records or reports as the employing organization was willing to make available.

It was in connection with the tracking of work experiences that an unanticipated advantage emerged from conducting the Work and Cancer studies serially. Several third-party employment reports, and especially in the dyads, had disclosed that decisions of some potential employers had been influenced by medical reports from the patients' physicians or the companies' own examining doctors. The two later studies, therefore, included additional areas of inquiry aimed at clarifying how the doctors' responses or reports influenced decisions about the patients' work. What did the doctor tell the inquiring employer about current or future employability of the patient? How and who in the doctor's office, and under what circumstances, released information—and what kinds—to the employer or to an insurance company? Would a statement emanating from the doctor or his office affect either the patient's or the employer's attitudes about the patient as a worker? In addition to those conducted with subsets of physicians for other study purposes, 25 percent of the doctors of consenting patients comprised this sample in the BC and YS studies.

Another possible source of enlightening data was incorporated in the BC study that was not included in the other two of the trilogy: labor unions. Interviews were conducted with officials of seven large unions represented among the occupations present in the BC study to learn if or how they assumed a role as protector or advocate of union members with cancer. Although some WC respondents had identified themselves as union members, none had mentioned the union as a source to which they turned for help or comfort when a work problem of any kind had arisen. Nor did BC respondents, a larger proportion (24 percent) of whom were union members, name the union or any official as a resource. But unlike the clues that led to productive inclusion of doctors in the later studies, interviews with union officials added no insights except to confirm what already had been inferred from the employee and employer interviews, namely: union contracts automatically protected individuals with cancer from being singled out from others in relation to employee benefits, salary adjustments, or job retention. No instance was reported by the union, employer, or employee of intercession on behalf of the individual patient who thought a work action was precipitated by the cancer history.

The degree of objectivity possible in establishing the validity of responses in a study as emotionally charged as one that couples cancer and work has definite limits, and from study to study there was renewed vigilance to optimize the objectivity and veracity of the data gathered. Language used by the research team was particularly scrutinized and selected. For example, at no time in employer or patient interviews were words used like "discrimination," "unfair," and "disability." Responses to queries about "changes," or "problems," and so on, were later classified into the problem categories defined in the next section. But did the fact that the focus of the studies was identified as *cancer* in some fashion consciously or subliminally affect attitudes or responses of the non-patients in the samples? With the passage of time, however, the validity of the methods described above has been reinforced, pragmatically experiential though they were. Subsequent events and observations affirmed incidents described by patients and confirmed by employers; subsequent events also reinforced the complexity and near impossibility of developing a faultless design that acknowledged the unique constellations and differences in personalities and perceptions among even closely related individuals—especially with regard to their work behavior and, hence, experiences.

Issues and Problems in Conducting Work and Cancer Research

As is likely in any multi-dimensional research dependent on human response about an emotion-filled condition, the course of the research described here was punctuated by some anticipated and some unexpected incidents and conditions. Several have been selected for comment here because of their generalizability to other efforts to examine psychosocial aspects of cancer-related work problems.

Patient-Sample Attrition

Attrition rates, because of some factors, exceeded expectations. The whereabouts of patients, averaging 24 percent per study, were no longer known. Less surprising was attrition among patients whose doctors or hospitals had authorized contact: from 23 percent (WC) to 35 percent (BC) failed to answer multiple letters. Most surprising, perhaps, was the number of physicians who withheld consent to contact patients because the latter did not know the diagnosis or the doctors did not want their patients "troubled" by researchers. It is also evident that some refusals of consent—or failure to respond—were related to the psychological and political climate in which the studies were instituted and conducted.

The Psychological and Political Climate

The Work and Cancer studies were carried out against a background of rising cost of medical malpractice insurance and increasing numbers of malpractice suits. Wide news media publicity had rendered physicians and hospitals particularly sensitive to outside inquiries about patient matters. Doctors, hospitals, and public interest groups increasingly were zealous about compliance with statutory and regulatory safeguards aimed at preserving confidentiality, guarding against invasion of privacy, and assuring that consent was truly informed. This zealousness was paralleled by uneasiness among some medical personnel and facilities about even agreeing that a patient might be approached with an invitation to decide for himself whether to participate in an interview.

Interviews with potential or actual employers also were affected by statutory and regulatory elements. The WC study was developed in an atmosphere of growing interest in affirmative action in general and federal and state statutory expectations in particular about employment of persons with handicaps or disabilities. California legislative interest was mounting about amending the Fair Employment Practices Act to protect "rehabilitated or cured" cancer patients form workplace discrimination (California Labor

Code 1977) and the youth project was being launched as the Federal Rehabilitation Act of 1973 became the target of considerable news coverage because of demonstrations by handicapped veterans protesting failure of the federal government to issue regulations to implement it.

Notwithstanding the proffered signed consent for release of information, key managerial personnel in some business firms were understandably wary about being interviewed, either about a named employee or applicant or about employment policies and practices in general. Some declined entirely, others were guarded in their responses; still others shared information freely. In either of the first two situations, unless the information sought was general and could be obtained in some other employment setting, effort was made to reach several persons at various hierarchical levels within the organization so that consistency of responses could serve at least as a partial guide to their accuracy. This strategem did indeed yield useful results. Not only did it disclose consistent or inconsistent interpretations of official organizational policies; it also highlighted the frequency of top management's unawareness of ways in which "gatekeepers" (examining physicians, job interviewers, personnel officers) might act against an employee or job applicant out of their personal views or fears about the individual's health history. On the other hand, it also underscored instances of management behavior allegedly to "reduce discomfort" among a returning employee's co-workers who, in turn, denied that *they* rather than the manager or supervisor were anxious about being in the presence of the person with the cancer experience.

Attitudes of Medical and Hospital Personnel

The roles of the physician as the patient's care-provider and as a policy maker or guider in the hospital that supplied the patient's care were especially significant in the trilogy of work studies and in the Greenleigh (1979) study; their effect on research undertakings on psychosocial aspects of cancer, particularly work-related activity, cannot be underestimated. Each role merits some separate attention here.

Earlier, the process was described for constructing the sample of patients, including hospital agreement to approach the doctors from whom permission would be sought to invite participation of patients in the respective study. The initial request for cooperation was sent to the administrator of each hospital identified as having had some patients that met the study criteria. A substantial proportion, often with the concurrence of the appropriate hospital research or medical committee, for various reasons readily supplied the permissions sought. One large teaching hospital, despite the urging of the principals in its own comprehensive cancer program, declined to be involved, specifying that at some future time it might want to engage in research that would involve the same patients.

Two quite different kinds of learning resulted form these varied experiences with hospitals. The first was reinforcement of the importance of allowing sufficient lead time to construct a sample of patients for psychosocial research that would not be under the hospital's direct auspices and confined to its current or former patients. It was not probable that the central issue was that these were patients with cancer, for committees in three hospitals, for example, had given almost perfunctory approval to written requests for cooperation in the two adult studies but their review of the protocols in the youth study were more probing. For the research team, the problems lay not in the matter of eliciting and explaining the nature of cooperation sought but, rather, the time spanned by the process. Most of the committees met monthly or every two or three months: arranging for time on a crowded agenda, especially when several committees had to make decisions contingent on the prior actions of other committees, might require six or more months. Alerted to this possible passage of time consumed in the WC study, care was taken in the subsequent studies to dispatch requests to these hospitals almost before other preliminary tasks were completed in developing the succeeding studies. Indeed, nearly two years passed before all the bases had been touched and the requisite approvals obtained for the youth study from a key hospital; the process was initiated as far as possible in advance of the start of that project without waiting for a computer count of the number of patients that might be suitable subjects but using instead informal estimates supplied by hospital personnel. The explanations offered by this hospital for the delays were couched in terms of cautious concern for the protection of the interests of the patients and doctors but it was evident also that hospital politics and internecine rivalries were operating.

The other learning was different in nature, unexpected in the frequency of its occurrence, and reflective of subsequent experiences with some physicians that posed some questions among the researchers as to the extent to which the expressed physician attitudes might affect the patients' own views of their work roles. This was the frank objection in some of the committee meetings—that the doctor or hospital should in any way be engaged in a study that went beyond consideration of the medical care required to support or participate in research looking at the patient's work life—which, after all, is outside the physician's interest or domain. When open voting took place with the author present (which was not always the case), some but not all of the vocal dissenters voted for cooperating with the research project.

The WC study disclosed that more than 12 percent of the doctors failed to respond at all to two letters and subsequent telephone calls; another nearly 8 percent offered no reason for their refusal to permit contact with designated patients. A medical consultant to the research team randomly and informally telephoned a dozen of these 51 doctors seeking clues for their nonresponse or denials. Four categories of answers were received: the doctor did not want to be "involved," the doctor was fearful about malpractice issues and preferred to say *nothing* to *anybody* about *any* patient, the patient's work had no bearing on the patient's health care, and the patient was unaware of his cancer diagnosis. Because of such replies the inquiries in the subsequent studies were broadened to include subsets of doctors to learn what and how the patient was told of the diagnosis, why the doctor did not respond to the research letters, and—as was discussed earlier—what information was given by the doctor or his representative to an inquiring employer or insurance representative.

Parenthetically it is worth noting that the research interviewers brought to the interview process certain qualities that in a number of instances not only elicited rich material responsive to the research aims, but also had a significant therapeutic effect. All of the interviewers were especially sophisticated about human behavior and highly skilled in working effectively with it; all had considerable research experience in the health field; and several were specialists in work with young people. The interview schedules called for structured as well as open-ended responses and it had been expected that each interview would consume about 90 minutes. Pilot interviews, however, had indicated that once the interviewer's notebook was closed, the respondent began to share freely anger, anxiety, and other feelings that appeared in some instances to have been bottled up for some time. This was especially a common occurrence among single persons and the youth study respondents. As good listeners and resourceful social workers, after the research interview had ended, the interviewers not infrequently referred respondents to sources for help they either had not known of or had not previously utilized. It was in the context of such post-interview sessions that anger with the physician—or at times with an allegedly "overprotective" parent—was brought to the interviewer's attention.

It was evident in a high proportion of the interviews in the three Work and Cancer studies that the doctors held the respect, confidence, and affection of patients who saw their physicians as benefactors, interested in the respondents' well-being. Yet even some of those most highly regarded by the patient-respondent sometimes saw only the patient's surface persona. For example, one doctor in a sample subset created to learn how and what the patient was told of the diagnosis and prognosis, said of a patient with permanent voice impairment following surgical treatment for throat cancer, "He took it very well; he is quite stoical." The patient, foreman for many years in a large plumbing manufacturing establishment, had been demoted two weeks after returning to work because, he told the research interviewer, his supervisor thought he could not control his subordinates with his "squeaky voice box." He had not wanted his admired doctor to think he "couldn't take it like the real man" his doctor thought he was and so he had not exposed to the doctor either his fear and distress on learning about his speech damage, or his apprehension about how to cope with this. This patient's almost successful suicide attempt was thwarted by his alert wife.

Table 2.1
Interviewers in Work and Cancer Trilogy

		Totals
		344
Patients		
WC	138	
BC	123	
YS	83	
Individuals in employing establishments		107
Employing establishments (from 1 to 10,000 + employees)		62
Physicians		87
Parents or guardians		28
School personnel		20

Source: Compiled by author.

In the context of the preceding, it is important to underscore that by and large most doctors approached seemed genuinely interested in these Work and Cancer studies. Aside from some patients referred specifically by certain doctors for the pilot phase of each study to test the interview instruments, several asked that certain of their patients be interviewed even though they did not fall into the systematically structured samples: The physicians thought either that their experiences were worth hearing about, or it would be helpful to the patient to be engaged in the research activity, or both.

SOME FINDINGS ABOUT WORK AND CANCER

The Interviewers

Table 2.1 shows the respondents interviewed in the course of the three Work and Cancer studies. All were in person, with the exception of doctors, who generally were interviewed by telephone. Table 2.1 included 36 dyads, 12 in each study comprising employees and as many of the actual or prospective employers of each as could be identified and reached. The school personnel interviewees were teachers, nurses, and counselors or others, generally selected because they had been identified by present or former students as knowing the situation reported by the YS respondent. In addition, unplanned and informal interviews were held with other persons: a spouse, adult, child, or lover who either was present at the interview with the respondent or arranged an office appointment with the interviewer later at the respondent's request.

Work Status at Interview

WC and BC respondents, and YS respondents who had any kind of work experience,[2] were queried about pre-cancer as well as post-cancer work and, also, about health history that preceded or followed the cancer experience. The aim was twofold: to identify clues to elements other than the cancer that either before or after the cancer diagnosis might have had a bearing on the individual's work life, and to learn how or if the kind or frequency or timing of other illnesses might have affected work experiences.

It will be recalled that a criterion for inclusion in the WC and BC samples was full-time employment when the cancer was discovered. At interview, approximately 90 percent of the WC respondents were working, nearly 80 percent of these still with the pre-cancer employer although some had left and then returned after finding that conditions were better for them with the former employer. Eight-two percent of the BC respondents were working at interview, a smaller proportion (69 percent) with the organization that employed them prior to the cancer diagnosis.

Some of the findings in the Greenleigh study (1979) seemed to resemble those in the BC study: 82 percent of those employed full or part-time at diagnosis were still working when interviewed in the Greenleigh study; 65 percent were with the pre-cancer employer. Yet the resemblance was more apparent than real, probably a function of the variations in the sample characteristics, for the Greenleigh study had not similarly differentiated its respondents by occupational classification, site, or age. Although there were many sicker respondents in the Greenleigh investigation, age alone might account for some of the differences. Two-thirds of the respondents in the BC and WC studies were over 46 but sample construction criteria precluded their being past 53 years old and so they were less likely than Greenleigh respondents either to have reached retirement age or to be in part-time work by choice. It is of interest to note in this context that the patients reported by Ganz et al. (Chapter 7, this volume) likewise tended to be an older group: The mean age for the more than 29 percent of the 320 patients who were working was nearly 55 years and for the nonworking respondents, nearly 60 years. Also, as in the Greenleigh study, sickness was more prevalent among the nonworking Ganz population than was true in the Work and Cancer trilogy.

The Work and Cancer respondents were work-able, in their own view and their medical overseers'. These respondents did not see themselves as having a disability or handicap—even if they used a prosthesis that enabled them to function normally. With rare exceptions, the 13 percent of the WC and 22 percent of the BC patients who were only partially employed at the time of interview, were seeking full-time work. In contrast to the Greenleigh respondents, most of the 11 percent of unemployed WC subjects and 15 percent of the nonworking BC respondents were actively trying to find work.

Positive Workplace Experience

Nearly two-thirds of the respondents reported positive experiences in their work life following the diagnosis. Employers and fellow workers were helpful in many ways, especially when the returnee had to adjust to rigors imposed by the medical regimen or depleted energy: Patients were relieved of certain difficult physical tasks until strength could be restored; work schedules were altered temporarily to accommodate treatment or other needs; equipment was modified to facilitate the returning employee's handling of work assignments (telephones, for example, for individuals with voice impairment); one corporation executive's chauffeur escorted an employee to and from medical treatment until the course was completed; and so on.

Work Problems

However, even respondents who described helpfulness of employers or fellow workers—or customers—frequently spoke of problems in their work life that they attributed to the cancer history: more than half of the white-collar subjects, more than four-fifths of the blue-collar respondents, and more than half the youth study respondents, whether as members of the labor force or as students. As a matter of fact, nearly 70 percent of all the respondents at interview reported their attempts to change jobs or occupations since the cancer was found, either because of unpleasant or unfair conditions they associated with attitudes about cancer or to advance themselves in some way. Many were still trying. Others had abandoned the efforts, discouraged by rejections they blamed on the cancer history or because of prospective loss or reduction in health or other employee group benefits. Among many, the *wish* for change, although not always translated into action, was a signal of work stress among a group who ordinarily might be regarded as fairly stable employees: 40 percent of all the respondents had been with the pre-cancer employer for more than 10 years, only a fifth for less than two years.

The work problems that the patients attributed to their cancer fell into three categories. One consisted of events involving *gross discrimination,* such as dismissal or demotion; denial of promotion or of a job or cost-of-living or other wage increase granted fellow workers; termination of, or exclusion from, health or life or retirement benefits; or alteration of other work conditions explained as due to the cancer (a nurse transferred to night duty so other staff need not be near her; a teacher shifted from classroom duties to "protect" her pupils).

A second category comprised attitudes encountered in the work environment that, though having common roots with the gross discrimination group, did not necessarily directly affect work hours, pay, benefits, or job retention. These *workplace attitudes* included avoidance or shunning by co-workers; overt hostility (mimicking the individual using a voice box); a supervisor constantly taunting the recovered patient to produce a quantity of work not expected of others and publicly criticizing this employee for not "carrying his weight." Also reported in this category as a problem of serious dimensions is the "never-ending cloying overprotectiveness" and solicitude fellow workers exhibit that constitute a constant and uncomfortable reminder that the work-able recovered patient's independence and adequacy are in question, as is his or her mortality.

The third category of work problems encompassed a constellation of *personal attitudes* of the respondent. These included such diverse attitudes as expectation that this individual's own negative longtime views toward others with cancer would now be directed toward the patient; discomfort about how to counter sympathy or avoidance by others; and self-imposed pressure shaped by lifelong work patterns established to demonstrate independence and productivity, to show "I'm still worth something!"; and others. Looming large within this category was a set of personal problems that undoubtedly interacted with personal attitudes like the aforementioned with the result that the depression and anger of the patient were deepened and, also, that they contributed to the negatives present in the workplace attitudes, if not to the actions categorized as discriminatory.

These personal problems evidenced by some adult respondents strongly resembled those that are often manifest in recently widowed persons, especially women: among others, rage, a sense of being abandoned, and a not uncommon unrealistic anxiety about economic security in their future. Such personal feelings sometimes were expressed as vulnerability to abandonment by others—their circle of friends in the workplace—and susceptibility to loss of earnings. It can be speculated that such feelings of anger, resentment, fear, depression, and other defensive mechanisms might interact in a variety of ways with the behaviors of others in the workplace and contribute to their exacerbation. The younger respondents also went through a mourning period, its intensity and duration affected by the operating developmental stage as, for example, facing loss of a body part to cancer during a life stage characterized by tremendous preoccupation with body image.

Various studies (Greenleigh 1979; Ganz, et al. [Chapter 7], this volume; Houts, et al. [Chapter 5], this volume) have commented on the importance to the patient of social supports. The Work and Cancer studies found that married respondents and those with close and loving support of lovers, families, and friends in the work environment were better able to cope with the exigencies of the illness and the situations that arose in relation to work. Accessible and caring physicians also were often instrumental in giving the patient support and courage to deal with return to the world of work. The role of social supports was especially valuable for students with pediatric cancers: Parents (particularly those with more education, higher incomes, and professional or managerial occupations), physicians, school personnel, and supportive peers were instrumental in encouraging the respondent to pursue educational and vocational interests and all provided emotional support in the process of coping with cancer-related problems that arose in the school or work arenas.

Many third-party interviews underscored the picture presented by the patient-respondent that problems in the work setting were connected with the cancer history, that sometimes the patient was helpless about coping with them except simply to accept them or try to move elsewhere. But not all. Some third-party interviews and from one to three dyads per study were at variance with the facts or interpretations offered by the patient-respondent. In one situation, for instance, the interviews disclosed long-standing personality problems that preceded the cancer: Quarrelsomeness and poor productivity led to the patient's separation form several successive pre-cancer jobs. Poor performance of another patient had resulted in a warning of dismissal several months before the patient's masectomy and resulted in firing six months later because her post-cancer performance had further deteriorated beyond a tolerable level. And some patients gained secondary benefits from using the diagnosis as an excuse not to work, claiming that special conditions required because of the cancer could not be met in proffered jobs. An example is the construction foreman who emphasized to prospective employers the necessity of having constant and immediate access to toileting facilities because of the cancer, a condition that none could promise to meet. The four potential employers confirmed this "obstacle," and the patient, who claimed to be the target of discrimination because of cancer, acknowledged to the employment interviewer that because he could not "find" work, he could devote his time to pursuit of a favored hobby.

In a different kind of situation, an employer reported that the patient, a waitress in a one-employee doughnut and coffee shop, regaled customers with intimate details of her surgery and treatments, refusing to heed warnings that she was driving away customers; the dismissed employee told the interviewer her employer thought cancer was "catching."

However the work problem was categorized—gross discrimination, or workplace, or personal attitudes—a significant thread bound them together. This was that in most of the reports of negative actions, the cause appeared not to be lessened productivity or efficiency, or absenteeism, or reluctance to keep or hire someone whose life expectancy would not justify the employer's investment in a job-training period, or poor past performance. Rather, the action seemed to emanate from the knowledge that the person in question had a history of cancer.

AUTHENTICATING FINDINGS OF WORK PROBLEMS

How valid are the findings about workplace problems of individuals with a cancer history, especially findings that allege gross discrimination? How have the findings in the Work and Cancer studies held up in the several years since the trilogy was completed?

When a reported problem, though described by the patient as "discrimination" or "unfair," was found to have been precipitated by the employee's behavior, it was classified under "work attitudes" or "personal attitudes" rather than as discrimination. Hence, the 25 percent of the WC–reported instances of gross discrimination, 43 percent of the BC–reported instances of gross discrimination, and 33 percent of the YC–reported incidents of workplace discrimination excluded alleged discriminatory actions that were refuted by the patients' own statements or by the third-party interviews, with or without documentation. Consequently, the above figures represent conservative findings.

It might be argued that the patterns discerned in the Work and Cancer studies about the nature and frequency of the occurrences do not really constitute evidence that discrimination has been practiced, or that problems in the workplace are necessarily connected with a cancer history because of attitudes about cancer held by people working in the employment establishment and even among patients themselves. But this argument is refutable if simply on the grounds that public views of cancer as contagious or a punishment for past transgressions are not credible just because they are widespread and identifiable; they merely reflect misinformation that calls for correction. The perceptions of negative workplace experiences reported in these studies, however, were confirmed in sufficient instances by the third-party interviews to give them credibility. Furthermore, subsequent formal and informal inquiries undertaken by the author as well as others tend to confirm the persistence of certain attitudes and experiences that impair the work opportunities and satisfactions of some people just because they have been treated for cancer.

Issues of Validation

The Work and Cancer trilogy disclosed that a substantial number of patient-respondents who performed their work sufficiently well to be retained in their jobs without any reference to the cancer history—or even despite it—were promoted, given salary raises and enlarged responsibility in the workplace; some patients, including several who reported cancer-related problems in the pre-cancer employment setting, were enticed away from the pre-cancer employer by others who had full knowledge of the cancer history. On the whole, patient-respondents for many reasons were reflected by some employer-respondents to have better records with respect to absenteeism than appeared the case with noncancer employees, and many behaved and were perceived as though the cancer had never been found.

Interestingly, the veracity of the *positive* reports has not had to be substantiated. They generally simply are taken as given. Yet, whenever the same patient describes good experiences and unfair or negative behavior in relation to his cancer history, the latter report provokes skepticism and proof must be provided to support any request for remedial action. Such expectations for evidenciary support hold special implications not just for the work-oriented recovered cancer patient, but also for research methodology in the psychosocial dimension of work and cancer. With regard to the former, already impaired self-esteem as well as psychological defense mechanisms undoubtedly accounted for the reluctance of some of the patients to confront individuals whose attitudes or actions they found stressful. In addition, the reduced self-esteem in tandem with an overwhelming sense of defeat because of the combination of work problems and cancer may explain why relatively few aggrieved employees have sought remedial action under California statutes designed to protect recovered cancer patients against discrimination in the workplace because of the cancer.

Toward a Precise Methodology

Elsewhere in this chapter some of the problems in designing and conducting psychosocial research that can yield incontrovertible data about the nature and degree of problems that appear in the workplace because of an individual employee's cancer history have been noted. Ideally, a study of work and cancer interrelationships would be longitudinal, following a large population over a period of years prior to and following onset of cancer, and tracking the before and after coping patterns of those with cancer and those who have had other serious illnesses—or none. There would be no need to artificially form matching samples for control or comparison purposes, for there is some reason to believe many of these are an exercise to provide form regardless of substance. Various devices might be employed to confirm cause and effect, to detect and analyze intrapersonal, interpersonal, and environmental elements operating to produce positive and negative outcomes.

A growing number of research activities in the last several years have been addressing the association of work problems with cancer histories. These do not lend themselves to ready comparison because the study populations and the methodologies are not sufficiently similar, and yet this researcher ventures to state that their findings do not need to be congruent to be compelling. In their different ways they have yielded clues to the existence of cancer-related work problems that should not be ignored. And the Work and Cancer studies have demonstrated a volume of confirmed discriminatory workplace actions along with other kinds of work problems—and satisfactions—that point to the significant impact of work on the quality of the lives of many recovered cancer patients and to the nature of their distress when work problems exacerbate the vulnerability to which they already have been subjected by the cancer itself.

Toward Precise Definitions

The experience in the Work and Cancer studies and the Greenleigh study, examination of other research directly or incidentally connecting the work and cancer experiences, review of actual and proposed state and federal legislation to protect recovered cancer patients from discrimination in the labor force, and scrutiny of some cases brought before the courts or workers' compensation bodies—all suggest that the absence of generally accepted definitions for certain critical words is an impediment to effective efforts to destigmatize the bringing of cancer histories into the workplace. What does "discrimination" mean? How can terms like "cured" or "recovered" or "disability" be explained in rules and regulations, and enter professional and common speech so that connotations that result have a reasonable degree of common meaning? It was found several times in the WC and BC studies, for example, that doctors hedged when asked by a prospective employer if an applicant's cancer was "cured." They balked at the term, telling the employer and confirming this with the researcher, that they could not *promise* that there would be no recurrence of cancer.

To develop terminology sufficiently precise yet flexible to guide researchers and thereby make their results useful to policy makers, helpful to employees, employers, and others is a difficult but necessary task. The importance of doing so might best be conveyed in the story told about Confucius. He was asked, "If the Prince of Wei were to ask you to take over the government, what would you put first on your agenda?" "The one thing needed," replied the Master, "is the definition of terms. If terms are ill-defined, statements disagree with facts; when statements disagree with facts, business is mismanaged; when business is mismanaged, order and harmony do not flourish, then justice becomes arbitrary; and when justice becomes arbitrary, the people do not know how to move hand or foot."

In order that all key "people" *will* know how to move hand and foot so that the quality of life of work-oriented persons with a history of cancer is not diminished because of attitudes in the work environment that derive from folklore and antiquity, research completed or now in progress should provide a basis both for developing useful definitions and for conducting further research that will illuminate how "hand and foot" can and should be moved.

NOTES

1. The first study was made possible in large measure because the limited funds were augmented by the voluntary contributions of a number of individuals and resources. In addition to the volunteer services of the principal investigators, resources were provided by the Cancer Surveillance Program of the University of Southern California's Comprehensive Cancer Center and the University's Computer

Center. Staff and faculty and alumni of the School of Social Work, University of Southern California made distinctive and important contributions to the conduct and completion of the trilogy, but especially the first of the group: the unexpected death of one of the principal investigators led the Dean and several faculty of the School to fill in the void that had thus occurred.

2. At interview, half of the YS respondents were in school and the other half were employed full or part-time. Twelve percent of the YS sample worked full-time while going full-time to high school or college. All the part-time workers also were going to school, either full- or part-time.

REFERENCES

Bettenson, H. S., ed. *Documents of the Christian church*, New York: Oxford University Press, 1947.

California Labor Code. Parts 4, 5, Fair Employment Practices, Sec. 1413(1), added by State, Chapter 1188, 1977.

Feldman F. L. *Work and cancer health histories: A study of experiences of recovered patients.* San Francisco: American Cancer Society, California Division, 1976.

Feldman, F. L. *Work and cancer health histories: A study of the experiences of recovered blue-collar workers.* San Francisco: American Cancer Society, California Division, 1978.

Feldman, F. L. *Work and cancer health histories: Work expectations and experiences of youth (ages 13–23) with cancer histories.* San Francisco: American Cancer Society, California Division, 1980.

Feldman, F. L., & Scherz, F. H. *Family social welfare: Helping troubled families.* New York: Aldine-Atherton Press, 1968.

Greenleigh Associates. *Report on the social, economic and psychological needs of cancer patients in California.* San Francisco: American Cancer Society, California Division, 1979.

McKenna, R. Analysis of case histories: Employability problems of the recovered cancer patient. San Francisco: American Cancer Society, Ad Hoc Committee, California Division, 1973.

Neff, W. S. *Work and human behavior.* New York: Aldine Publishing Company, 1985.

O'Toole, J. *Work in America.* Cambridge, MA: MIT Press, 1973.

Stone, R. W. Employing the recovered cancer patient. *Cancer*, 1975 (suppl.), *36*, 285–286.

Tawney, R. H. *Religion and the rise of capitalism.* New York: Harcourt, Brace, 1926.

Weber, M. *The Protestant ethic and the spirit of capitalism.* London: Allen and Unwin, 1930.

Wheatley, G. M., Cunnick, W. R., Wright, B. P., & Van Deuren, D. The employment of persons with a history of treatment for cancer. Metropolitan Life Insurance Company Study. *Cancer*, 1974, *33*, 441–445.

3

Socioeconomic Sequelae of Childhood and Adolescent Cancer Survival

M. Jane Teta

INTRODUCTION

As recently as the 1960s a medical text characterized pediatric cancer as "a seemingly insoluble human problem" (Schiefelbein 1981). Fifteen to 20 years ago the prospects were dim for surviving childhood cancer. Recent advances in medicine, however, have dramatically improved this picture—to the point where 50 percent of newly diagnosed childhood cancer patients can expect to live for many years. For example, since 1967 the survival rate for patients diagnosed with Wilms' tumor has risen from 49 percent to 80 percent; with acute lymphocytic leukemia, from 20 percent to 60 percent; with non-Hodgkin's lymphoma, from 40 percent to 70 percent. In the 1960s, only 5 percent to 20 percent of young patients with osteogenic sarcoma, a bone cancer, survived; today, in top U. S. cancer centers, as many as 80 percent of such patients survive (Schiefelbein 1981). Indeed, by 1990, an estimated one of every 1000 adults will be a survivor of childhood cancer (Meadows & Silber 1985).

These figures have helped to establish pediatric cancer victims as individuals for whom quality of life issues, beyond the purely physiological, become important components of their long-term prognosis. Many survivors of childhood cancer now reach adulthood, marry, have offspring, and desire active participation in society. As a result of public attitudes, individual fears, physical limitations, and other consequences of surviving a life-threatening illness, however, their ability to attain major socioeconomic goals may be compromised.

With the availability of increased numbers of adult childhood cancer survivors, researchers have begun to investigate the impact of this disease experience on their lives. Holmes and Holmes (1975) posed the question, "After ten years, what are the handicaps and the life styles of children treated for cancer?" These authors' examination of the present status of 124 survivors, known to be alive from the Tumor Registry of the University of Kansas Medical Center, marked a milestone in chronic illness research. The researchers examined current physical problems, any history of subsequent cancer, disability, education, employment, and marital status, and even current attitudes toward the childhood disease experience. It was reported in this investigation that 69 percent of the survivors had completed high school, 15 percent were attending high school, 19 percent were attending or had graduated from college. The average age at high school graduation was 17.8 years, equivalent to that expected. Eleven percent were school dropouts, after the exclusion of seven, who suffered severe disabilities as a result of brain tumors. Although no control group was included in this investigation, the educational and vocational achievements of study subjects were judged to be comparable to those of their parents.

A similar though more formal study used a registry of patients established at the Sidney Farber Cancer Center, Boston, to examine, with a medical record review and questionnaire survey, the late effects of childhood cancer in 142 former patients presently aged 18 years and over (Li & Stone 1976). Of this cohort, 86 (69%) had attended college and 36 (29%) were employed as professionals or managers. The illness and its treatment did not appear to delay their education. Individual patients, however, reported that because of their history of cancer they experienced difficulty obtaining permanent employment or job-related insurance benefits.

A comprehensive effort to investigate consequences of surviving childhood cancer is reflected in the work of Koocher and O'Malley (1981). As with the work of Li and Stone (1976), the Sidney Farber Cancer Registry was used to identify children and adolescents diagnosed with cancer between 1948 and 1970, who were less than 18 years of age at diagnosis and survived at least five years. The book reports on 117 selected former patients, ranging from five to 30 years in age—and their families—who were studied and interviewed in this extensive survey. Intellectual functioning, social maturity, depression, death anxiety, and relationship to overall adjustment were assessed. Several social issues or concerns were also identified by Koocher and O'Malley (1981) as existing for childhood cancer survivors. These included the effects of physical impairment, employment discrimination, and insurance problems. The analyses of these outcomes were limited to the 60 of the 117 patients in the sample who were over 18 years of age at the time of the interview. It was reported that 62 percent had completed some education beyond high school while 5 percent were not high school graduates. Seventy-seven percent were working at the time of the interview. One was still a full-time high school student and had never applied for a job. Some form of employment discrimination because of a history of cancer was reported by 40 percent (24). This included 11 who were rejected for military service. Absenteeism on the job was low in this sample. Of the 46 employed former patients, 43 missed work fewer than five days during the previous year, two were absent from six to 15 days, and only one was absent for 16 days or more. Some of the survivors reported that they had never informed their employers of their medical history.

At the time of interview, 87 percent of these former patients were covered by some form of health insurance, but more than 10 percent reported problems in obtaining this coverage because of their cancer history. Sixty-three percent of these individuals had some form of life insurance at the time of interview, although nine had a policy that was obtained on their behalf before the cancer was diagnosed. Forty-two percent reported being denied a life insurance policy at least once, 13 percent had been asked to pay a higher premium than usual and 10 percent were required to wait from three to 12 years after diagnosis before they would be granted a life insurance policy. Overall, two-thirds of the recovered childhood cancer patients in this study believe they had experienced discrimination in their attempts to obtain employment, health insurance, or life insurance, solely because of their history of cancer.

These early attempts to examine psychosocial consequences of childhood cancer survival were limited by small numbers, the absence of control populations, and failure formally to assess the possible contributions of clinical factors related to the cancer diagnoses. They did succeed, however, in raising the issue that survivors of childhood cancer may face impediments in their quest for insurance and employment as a result of their medical history.

The NCI Childhood and Adolescent Cancer Study

In 1981, the National Cancer Institute (NCI) initiated a five-center study to examine the occurrence of second primaries, infertility, birth defects in offspring, and occupational and educational characteristics of long-term survivors of childhood and adolescent cancer. Study subjects, identified for inclusion from the registrants of tumor registries in five states, were diagnosed at age 19 or younger, between 1945 and 1974, with a histologically confirmed malignant neoplasm or any brain tumor, and survived five years or more to reach at least age 21 by December 31, 1979.

Interviews were conducted in-person whenever possible, and by telephone under special circumstances (subject now living out-of-state, subject's desire not to share disease experience information with other family members, etc.), by NCI–trained staff. The main components of the NCI questionnaire concerned educational and occupational history, personal health, reproductive history, children's health status, and health of other family members. The most knowledgeable available proxy was selected when respondents were deceased, incompetent, or unavailable for the interview.

The Connecticut component of this multi-center study was conducted by the Connecticut Cancer Epidemiology Unit of the Yale University School of Medicine, the research affiliate of the Connecticut Tumor Registry (CTR), the oldest population-based tumor registry in the United States. An addendum to the main NCI questionnaire, which addressed depression, insurability, and the frequency of rejection for military, educational, and occupational goals was administered in Connecticut. The Connecticut Addendum was developed in response to the psychological and socioeconomic needs of pediatric cancer survivors, as expressed by the Connecticut and national leadership of the Candelighters Foundation, a support group for parents of children with cancer. The Connecticut Addendum was administered only to eligible study subjects themselves. Proxies were excluded because the Addendum questions could be readily and reliably answered only by the actual study subject.

The occurrence of a definite major depressive syndrome (DMDS), either current or past, among respondents to the Addendum was identified by an abbreviated psychological interview, based on a modified version of the schedule of affective disorders (SADS-L; Spitzer, et al. 1978; Endicott & Spitzer 1978). The findings, which have been described elsewhere in greater detail, did not suggest any greater frequency of depression among long-term childhood cancer survivors than among their siblings, with the exception of women who survived genital cancers, who were eight times more likely to have experienced a major depression (Teta, et al. 1986).

The second portion of the Addendum queried whether respondents had ever applied for the military, college, employment, health insurance, and life insurance. Those who answered affirmatively were asked whether they were ever rejected, and if so, their perceptions of the reason for denial. Interviewers were carefully trained not to probe study subjects differentially or suggest in any way the issue of discrimination.

Permission was sought from interviewed survivors in all five states to contact their siblings to be interviewed as members of the study's comparison group. Up to two full siblings, who were born before December 31, 1960, and survived to at least 19 years of age, were selected. Preference was given to siblings of the same sex and closest in age to the case.

The choice of sibling controls was motivated by the intent to maximize participation and to adjust efficiently for a large number of potential confounders—for example, social class, genetic background, ethnicity, religion—which would be difficult otherwise to incorporate into the study design. Since siblings themselves may have been affected by the disease experience, they do not constitute a "pure" control population. Differences observed for outcomes such as educational and occupational status may be an underestimate of the true impact of childhood cancer survival.

Both matched and unmatched analyses were conducted. For the matched analyses, each matched pair consisted of a survivor and one sex-matched sibling. This necessitated the exclusion of cases who either had no same sex siblings, or their same sex siblings were ineligible, or for some other reason did not participate. For survivors who had two sibling participants, the same sex sibling closest in age was selected. Parallel unmatched analyses were conducted when: (1) there was reasonable concern that the results may have been influenced by the reduction in sample size due to the exclusion of survivors with no siblings or no same sex siblings or (2) it was appropriate to conduct internal comparisons, using the population of survivors only in an attempt to identify clinical factors (tumor type, age at diagnosis, treatment type, etc.) predictive of adverse outcomes in the survivor population. The odds ratio (OR) was utilized where appropriate and easily interpretable as the measure of relative risk. In the context of this investigation, it represented the odds of an occurrence among survivors compared to the odds among their brothers and sisters.

Sample Characteristics

Five Center Population

Of the 2644 identified survivors of childhood cancer from the five participating centers, 146 were declared ineligible upon examination of hospital records and another 215 were not interviewed for an overall nonresponse rate of 9 percent. The 2498 eligible subjects included 296 deceased cases, 256 (86%) of whom were interviewed by proxy. Table 3.1 describes the eligible survivor population by primary site group. The largest categories were survivors of Hodgkin's disease (547), brain tumors (371), and soft tissue sarcoma (312).

A total 3261 siblings were interviewed of 3606 who were eligible (90% response rate) together with 2283 cases for a total interviewed sample size of 5544. The mean age for cases was 31 years (S.D. = 6.6); for siblings it was 33 years (S.D. = 7.8). Ninety percent of the study population was white.

Of the 2283 survivors interviewed, 1453 had at least one sibling of the same sex interviewed. There were 716 male and 737 female sibling matched pairs for the pooled analyses. Seventy-five percent of the pairs were within ± five years of age, with a maximum difference of 37 years.

Connecticut Population

Of the 643 eligible CT survivors of childhood cancer (see Table 3.1), 534 (83%) were interviewed for the NCI portion of the study. They provided

Table 3.1
Childhood and Adolescent Cancer Survivors by Primary Site

Primary Site	Connecticut	Five Centers
Leukemia	15	49
Hodgkin's Disease	142	547
Non-Hodgkin's Lymphoma	41	131
Brain	96	371
Neuroblastoma	23	55
Soft Tissue Sarcoma	80	312
Kidney	24	56
Bone	32	145
Retinoblastoma	21	62
Thyroid Gland	42	235
Melanoma of the Skin	30	110
Female Genital	29	118
Male Genital	16	78
Other	61	229
Total	643	2,498

Source: Compiled by author.

847 eligible controls, of whom 736 (87%) were interviewed. Connecticut, therefore, conducted 1270 total interviews for an overall response rate of 85 percent.

The Connecticut Addendum questions were asked only of subjects themselves. The exclusion of proxy respondents left 445 survivors to whom the Addendum could be administered. Of the 669 nonproxy sibling interviews, 92 were excluded as siblings of survivors interviewed by proxy. There were, then, 577 sibling addenda and 445 survivor addenda for a total of 1022.

Results: NCI Questionnaire

Occupational Performance

Based on the pooled five-center data, analysis of employment status for males revealed that almost twice as many survivors were unemployed at the time of interview (19% vs. 10%) and 20 male survivors had never worked as opposed to three siblings (Table 3.2). The male survivor and sibling distributions across the three levels of employment (full-time, part-

Table 3.2
Current Employment Status of Five Center Study Subjects[1] by Sex

	SURVIVORS (%)	SIBLINGS (%)	X^2*(P VALUE)
MALES			
EMPLOYED FULL-TIME	459(73)	533(85)	
EMPLOYED PART-TIME	51(8)	32(5)	
NOT EMPLOYED AT ALL	116(19)	61(10)	
NEVER EMPLOYED	20	3	29.37(0.00)
	626(100)	626(100)	
FEMALES			
EMPLOYED FULL-TIME	304(47)	320(50)	
EMPLOYED PART-TIME	102(16)	110(17)	
NOT EMPLOYED AT ALL	238(37)	214(33)	
NEVER EMPLOYED	32	20	2.06(0.15)
	644(100)	644(100)	

[1] Number of matched pairs excludes those administered version 1 of questionnaire which did not distinguish part-time from full-time employment.

* Stuart-Maxwell Chi-square Statistic on 2 df.

Source: Compiled by author.

time, not employed) were statistically different (p = 0.00). The female distributions, however, were more similar (p = 0.15) with 37 percent and 33 percent unemployed, respectively. Thirty-two female survivors had never worked versus 20 sisters in this category.

When the annual income levels of employed study subjects were examined, male survivors appeared to have a larger proportion of individuals in the lower income categories (Table 3.3). Twelve percent more were earning under $15,000 per year and 5 percent fewer were earning $25,000–50,000 per year. The Chi-square test rejected the hypothesis of homogeneity of proportions (p = 0.00). Females evidenced a suggestion of lower income levels, but the differences were not significant (p = 0.07).

Respondents reported study subjects' most recent job category as one of the following: farming, skilled labor, unskilled labor, professional (health), professional (other), clerical, or managerial. For analysis, these were reduced to four groups: managerial and professional, skilled labor, clerical, and unskilled labor. Farmers were categorized as skilled labor. Tables 3.4 and 3.5 present the distributions of male and female study subjects by these four

Table 3.3
Annual Income[1] of Employed Five Center Study Subjects by Sex

	SURVIVORS (%)	SIBLINGS (%)	X^2(P VALUE)
MALES			
15	288(44)	207(32)	
15-24	217(33)	260(40)	
25-50	120(18)	152(23)	
50+	29(5)	35(5)	27.85(0.00)
	654(100)	654(100)	
FEMALES			
15	483(75)	465(72)	
15-24	139(21)	151(23)	
25-50	23(4)	29(4)	
50+	3(0)	3(0)	3.30(0.07)
	648(100)	648(100)	

[1] In thousands of dollars.

*Stuart-Maxwell Chi-square Statistic on 2 df, collapsing highest two income levels into 25+.

Source: Compiled by author.

Table 3.4
Most Recent Job Description of Employed Male Five Center Study Subjects

	SURVIVORS (%)	SIBLINGS (%)	$\bar{R}$(se)*	P Z (VALUE)
MANAGERIAL & PROFESSIONAL	298(44)	350(51)		
SKILLED LABOR	254(36)	268(39)		
CLERICAL	33(5)	19(3)		
UNSKILLED LABOR	104(15)	49(7)	0.57(0.01)	7.00(0.00)
	686(100)	686(100)		

*$\bar{R}$(se) = mean ridit and standard error.
Source: Compiled by author.

Table 3.5
Most Recent Job Description of Employed Female Five Center Study Subjects

	SURVIVORS (%)	SIBLINGS (%)	R̄(se)*	Z	P (VALUE)
MANAGERIAL & PROFESSIONAL	278(42)	304(46)			
SKILLED LABOR	73(11)	79(12)			
CLERICAL	225(34)	194(29)			
UNSKILLED LABOR	89(13)	88(13)	0.52(0.01)	2.00(0.04)	
	665(100)	665(100)			

*R̄(se) = mean ridit and standard error.
Source: Compiled by author.

job categories. Ridit analyses indicated statistically significant different proportions for both sex groups with a male survivor mean ridit of 0.57 and a female survivor mean ridit of 0.52. Thus, male survivors appeared to be 33 percent (0.57/0.43) more likely to be in lower occupational positions than their brothers and females appeared 8 percent (0.52/0.48) more likely to be in lower level positions than their sisters. Both survivor groups had fewer members in the highest level (managerial and professional). More males survivors were in the lowest category (unskilled labor). An equal percentage (13%) of female survivors and siblings belonged to the unskilled labor category. Job tenure was also shorter for survivors of both sex groups and the differences were statistically significant.

Survivors also reported that their health problems affected their ability to work more often than did siblings (Table 3.6). For males these included problems related to hearing ($\hat{O}R$ = 2.4), vision ($\hat{O}R$ = 3.0), emotional problems ($\hat{O}R$ = 1.6), and general health ($\hat{O}R$ = 3.6). Female relative odds were also elevated for these outcomes, although emotional problems were not as evident ($\hat{O}R$ = 1.1) as in the male comparison. These findings were also observed when cases were restricted to survivors who were diagnosed (and presumably under treatment) prior to age 16 and the commencement of their work experience. Eighty-five percent of the survivors (vs. 92 percent of siblings) described their health as excellent or good, while 3 percent (vs. 1% for siblings) said it was poor (Table 3.7).

An internal comparison within the survivor population was conducted to assess possible associations between age at diagnosis, primary site and treatment modality, with current employment status (working vs. not working), while simultaneously controlling for the potential confounding of sex, race, and years of education for the cases' fathers (the surrogate measure for social class) (Table 3.8). The only extraneous covariate which

Table 3.6
Factors Affecting Ability to Work by Sex: Five Center Study Subjects

FACTOR	MALES (N = 716)					FEMALES (N = 737)				
	S /B yes no	S /B¹ no yes	X* MH	P VALUE	ÔR (95% CI)	S /Sr² yes no	S /Sr no yes	X MH	P VALUE	ÔR (95% CI)
HEARING	17	7	1.84	0.07	2.4(0.9,7.3)	18	3	3.05	0.00	6.0(1.5,36.7)
VISION	54	18	4.12	0.00	3.0(1.7,5.5)	41	18	2.86	0.00	2.3(1.2,4.3)
EMOTIONAL PROBLEMS	45	28	1.87	0.06	1.6(1.0,2.7)	49	43	0.52	0.60	1.1(0.7,1.8)
GENERAL HEALTH	189	53	8.68	0.00	3.6(2.6,5.0)	161	46	7.92	0.00	3.5(2.5,5.0)

*Cannot be calculated. Division by zero.
¹Survivor yes, brother no.
²Survivor yes, sister no.
*Mantel-Haenszel Test for matched pairs (McNemar's Test).

Source: Compiled by author.

Table 3.7
Perceived Health Status of Five Center Study Subjects[1] by Sex

HEALTH STATUS	MALE		FEMALE	
	SURVIVORS(%)	SIBLINGS(%)	SURVIVORS(%)	SIBLINGS(%)
EXCELLENT	240(43)	286(51)	261(42)	314(50)
GOOD	244(43)	238(42)	266(43)	253(41)
FAIR	59(10)	36(6)	81(13)	49(8)
POOR	21(4)	4(1)	15(2)	7(1)
	564(100)	564(100)	623(100)	623(100)

[1] Proxy interviews excluded.

Source: Compiled by author.

Table 3.8
Adjusted Odds Ratios for Variables Significantly Related[1] to Employment Status[2] Among Survivors from Five Centers

Variable	$\hat{OR}$	95% CI
Sex (female/male)	0.30	(0.2, 0.4)
Treatment Modality:		
Chemotherapy + Radiation/Surgery	0.48	(0.4, 0.6)
Radiation/Surgery	0.74	(0.6, 1.0)
Primary Site:		
Brain/Melanoma + Thyroid	0.25	(0.2, 0.3)

[1] Variables failing to enter the model (0.05 level for entry) were age at diagnosis (<15, ≥ 15 years); current age; number of years of education for father; race (white/nonwhite); and 11 other primary site subgroups.
[2] Currently employed or unemployed at time of death vs. not so employed.

Source: Compiled by author.

remained in the unconditional logistic model after fast backward elimination was sex. (Females were 70% less likely ($\hat{OR}$ = 0.30) to be employed than males.) Age at diagnosis showed no relationship with current job status. When compared to those receiving surgery alone, two other treatment groups had relatively fewer persons employed at time of interview. Those receiving radiation and chemotherapy were 52 percent less likely to be working ($\hat{OR}$ = .48), while the deficit for those receiving radiation without chemotherapy was 26 percent ($\hat{OR}$ = .74). The only primary site group which remained in the model was brain tumor. Survivors of this disease were 75 percent less likely to be employed ($\hat{OR}$ = 0.25, 95% CI: 0.2, 0.3) than the comparison subgroup of melanoma and thyroid cancer survivors combined.

Educational Performance

The results of the analysis of educational characteristics based on the pooled population of 1453 matched pairs are presented in Tables 3.9 and 3.10. Male survivors completed an average of 13.4 years of school compared

Table 3.9
Educational Characteristics of Five Center Study Subjects by Sex: Comparison of Means

| | MALES | | | | | FEMALES | | | |
FACTOR	N	SURVIVORS	SIBLINGS	PAIRED[1] T	P VALUE	N	SURVIVORS	SIBLINGS	PAIRED T	P VALUE
Number of years in school	714	13.4	13.6	-2.0	0.04	734	13.2	13.2	-0.03	0.97
Age at High School Graduation	546	17.8	17.8	-0.8	0.44	572	17.6	17.6	0.59	0.56
Age at Completion of schooling among those not completing high school	45	16.0	16.3	-0.9	0.40	48	15.6	15.6	0.11	0.91

[1] Student's T test for paired samples.

Source: Compiled by author.

Table 3.10
Educational Characteristics of of Five Center Study Subjects by Sex: Binary Outcomes

	MALES (N = 716)					FEMALES (N = 737)				
OUTCOME	S /B[1] yes no	S /B no yes	X* MH	P VALUE	$\widehat{OR}$(95% CI)	S /Sr[2] yes no	S /Sr no yes	X MH	P VALUE	$\widehat{OR}$ (95% CI)
Completion of 8th Grade	8	22	2.37	0.02	0.36(0.1,0.9)	7	12	0.92	0.36	0.58(0.2,1.8)
High School Completion	46	63	1.53	0.13	0.73(0.5,1.1)	50	63	1.13	0.26	0.79(0.5,1.2)
High School Drop-out	46	47	0.00	1.00	0.98(0.6,1.5)	53	49	0.30	0.77	1.08(0.7,1.7)
Completion of College	95	96	0.00	1.00	0.99(0.7,1.3)	79	76	0.16	0.87	1.04(0.7,1.5)

[1] Survivor yes, brother no.
[2] Survivor yes, sister no.
* Mantel-Haenszel Test for matched pairs (McNemar's Test).

Source: Compiled by author.

to 13.6 years for their brothers. This difference of two tenths of a year was statistically significant, however (p = 0.04). For females the averages were 13.2 for both survivors and for their sisters. The mean ages at high school graduation were also between 17.6 and 17.8 years old.

Thirty-nine survivors compared to 20 siblings did not complete eighth grade (Table 3.10). The difference in the total number of high school drop-outs, however, was smaller (160 vs. 157) and not significant for either sex group. Survivors of brain tumor (N = 213) accounted for 18 (46%) of the 39 cases who did not complete eighth grade. None of their matched siblings completed fewer than eight years of schooling. Twice as many male brain tumor survivors (30) did not achieve parity with their fathers as compared to their brothers (15). Female brain tumor survivors and their sisters differed only slightly, however, when their educational achievements were compared to that of their mothers.

On the average, survivors exceeded the educational levels of their parents. The approximate two-year mean differences were highly significant (p = 0.00). There were 149 male survivors (21%) and 119 female survivors (16%) who did not achieve parity with their same sex parent, compared to 18 percent and 17 percent of their brothers and sisters, respectively. The test of homogeneity of survivor and sibling proportions less than, equal to and exceeding parents' educational achievements was not statistically significant (males X^2_2 = 2.70, p= 0.26; females X^2_2 = 0.56, p= 0.76).

Multiple linear regression was employed to formally test the effects of primary site, age at diagnosis (<15, ≥15 years), physical impairments (Y/N) and treatment modality, adjusting for sex, race (white, nonwhite), and social class on educational achievement. Father's level of education again served as a surrogate measure for social class. A backward elimination procedure resulted in a model which included the terms described in Table 3.11. The regression was significant (F = 66.7 on 7, 2016 df, p = 0.00) with an R^2 of 0.19. Number of years of education was highly correlated with the highest level achieved by fathers and with age at time of interview. Age of diagnosis failed to enter the final model. Radiation with or without chemotherapy was inversely related to educational outcome. The diagnosis of a brain tumor was also inversely correlated (regression coefficient = -1.55, p = 0.00) and females achieved lower levels than males.

Results: Connecticut Addendum

There was substantial evidence from these data that male long-term survivors of childhood cancer had experienced significantly more rejection from the armed forces, undergraduate college, and employment than had siblings (Table 3.12). Based on the numbers who applied, which did not differ proportionately for the two groups, 80 percent of male survivors were rejected from the military vs. 18 percent of male siblings (p < 0.0001);

Table 3.11
**Variables Significantly Related[1] to Number of Years of Education
Completed by Survivors from Five Centers**

Variable	B Value	S.E.[2]	F[3] (p Value)
Fathers Years of Education	0.28	0.02	345.6(0.00)
Handicapped	-0.31	0.16	3.8(0.05)
Primary Site: Brain	-1.55	0.17	80.0(0.00)
Treatment Modality: Chemotherapy & Radiation	-0.38	0.17	4.8(0.03)
Radiation Only	-0.27	0.13	4.3(0.04)
Age	0.03	0.01	12.0(0.00)
Sex	-0.25	0.12	4.3(0.04)

[1] Variables not included in the final model (0.10 level of significance to stay) were race (white/nonwhite); age at diagnosis (<15, ≥15 years); treatment modalities (chemo only); 11 other primary site subgroups.

[2] S.E. = Standard Error.

[3] df for partial F tests = 1, 2016.

Source: Compiled by author.

for college admissions the proportions were 13 percent and 3 percent respectively (p < 0.01). The differences with respect to employment were also significant (p < 0.05) but not as disparate (32% vs. 21%). Of those male survivors with observable physical limitations (blindness, deafness, mobility problems, any deformity, other), 41 percent reported rejection from employment.

In contrast to the male differential, equal percentages of female survivors and siblings, 19 percent, were denied employment. The percentage denied employment among females with physical limitations, however, was much higher at 33 percent. Female survivors were also significantly more likely to be denied entrance into the military (p < 0.05). This association was based on a total of only 16 female study subjects who ever applied. The percentages of applicants for the military, college, or employment among females did not differ by disease status.

Although the differences were not significant, there appeared to be less rejection from graduate school among survivors of both sexes than among siblings, as well as significantly more graduate school applicants in the male survivor cohort (23%) than in the male sibling cohort (14%).

Table 3.12

Percentages of Survivor and Sibling Applicants Denied Military, Educational and Occupational Opportunities by Sex

	M A L E		F E M A L E	
	SURVIVORS	SIBLINGS	SURVIVORS	SIBLINGS
MILITARY	80 (92)[1]	18 (130)	75 (8)	13 (8)
P <	0.0001		0.05	
COLLEGE	13 (128)	3 (163)	6 (124)	7 (161)
P <	0.01		NS[2]	
GRADUATE SCHOOL	6 (47)	11 (38)	0 (30)	4 (46)
P <	NS		NS	
JOB	32 (210)	21 (267)	19 (224)	19 (299)
P <	0.05		NS	

[1]Number of applicants in parentheses.

[2]NS = Not Significant.

Source: Compiled by the author.

Both male and female survivors experienced denial of life insurance and health insurance more frequently than siblings (Table 3.13). The differences observed were highly significant. Based on the numbers who applied, 24 percent of male survivors and 29 percent of female survivors were denied life insurance; 14 percent of male survivors and 9 percent of female survivors were denied health insurance, in contrast to a negligible number of siblings denied insurance of either type. Survivors with physical limitations experienced a higher rate of rejection of life insurance (30% males; 37% females) than survivors without such handicaps. There were no apparent differences in the frequency of denial of health insurance, however.

The vast majority of insurance denials and rejections from the military were attributed by the respondents to reasons of health (Table 3.14). Although this information was not systematically collected, survivors reported waiting periods, waivers in policies, high premiums, and often the intercession of their physicians before being granted insurance. Others applying for mortgages were unable to obtain life insurance coverage as part of their mortgage agreement. Rejected applicants from graduate school did not feel that denial was due to their medical status. There were two areas in which significantly more survivors perceived rejection to be related to

Table 3.13
Percentages of Survivor and Sibling Applicants Denied Life and Health Insurance by Sex

	M A L E		F E M A L E	
	SURVIVORS	SIBLINGS	SURVIVORS	SIBLINGS
LIFE INSURANCE	24 (157)[1]	3 (200)	29 (141)	1 (163)
p <	0.0001		0.0001	
HEALTH INSURANCE	14 (114)	1 (147)	9 (98)	0 (112)
p <	0.0001			0.01

[1]Number of applicants in parentheses.

Source: Compiled by the author.

Table 3.14
Percentages of Survivor and Sibling Rejections Attributed to Medical History

		Percent Attributed to Medical History		
	N[1]	Survivors (%)	N	Siblings (%)
Military	80	95	31	100
College	24	17	17	0
Graduate School	3	0	6	0
Employment	109	46	115	9
Life Insurance	79	95	7	75
Health Insurance	25	84	2	100

[1]N = Number rejected

Source: Compiled by the author.

their medical history than did siblings. Seventeen percent of survivors and and no siblings felt their application to a college was rejected for reasons related to their past health. More than five times as many survivors (46%) than siblings (9%) perceived employment rejections to be related to their illness. The percentage was even higher for the physically handicapped survivors (54%).

A significant association was observed between having experienced a major depression and having been denied employment for both survivors and siblings. The estimated relative risk for survivors (1.98) was 14 percent higher than that for siblings (1.73). No association with depression was indicated for survivors denied life or health insurance, however.

Discussion

Education and Occupational Achievements

Overall, the educational accomplishments of survivors are not strikingly different from those of controls. This finding is consistent with the earlier reports of smaller populations (Holmes & Holmes 1975; Li & Stone 1976; Koocher & O'Malley 1981). There was an excess risk for failure to complete eighth grade, which was statistically significant for males. This was mainly attributable to educational deficits among male brain tumor survivors (Duffner et al. 1985). When this primary site was excluded from the analysis the odds ratio for completion of eighth grade among males was 0.73 but no longer statistically significant. There were nine female survivors who did not complete eighth grade, fewer than the number of siblings (11), after the exclusion of brain tumor survivors. Female educational achievements overall are very close to expectation. Males had on average 0.2 years less education than controls, which was statistically significant. This small difference was also influenced by the experience of brain tumor survivors.

Survivors' educational achievements, given the completion of eighth grade, are comparable to those of their siblings. They (and siblings) exceeded the educational levels of their parents by about two years. The proportions of survivors and siblings whose years of schooling were less than, equal to, or greater than parents did not differ. Again male brain tumor survivors were less likely to achieve parental parity.

In contrast to educational achievement, however, the occupational status of long-term survivors of childhood cancer appears to be less favorable than that of their siblings, particularly for males. A variety of measures including whether currently or ever employed; level of income, if employed; job skill level; and tenure in job held the longest suggested poorer performance for male survivors compared to their brothers. Female survivors, on the other hand, do not demonstrate such obvious differences. They also exhibited significantly shorter mean job tenure and lower skill levels in current occupations and showed a slight tendency toward less success in the other areas examined, when compared to their sisters.

Although brain tumor survivors were readily distinguishable from other cancer survivors by being only 25 percent as likely to be employed, they did not entirely explain the occupational patterns observed among male cases. Nor did the experience of those cases who ultimately died. This elimination did close the gap further among female cases and their sisters who were already quite comparable. Job tenure among females was no greater for siblings than for surviving cases. Individuals who had received radiation alone and combined chemotherapy and radiation were less likely to be employed at time of interview or at time of death than the comparison group of persons undergoing surgery only. These treatment-related associations were observed after adjustment for sex and primary site. Age at diagnosis did not appear related to employment status after adjustment for the other important covariates.

Employability and Insurability

The reasons for employment-related difficulties among male long-term survivors of childhood cancer are difficult to disentangle. These problems are consistent with perceived patterns of job rejections reported by survivors in the Connecticut Addendum, raising the issue of employment discrimination. Koocher and O'Malley (1981) reported a 40 percent rate of employment discrimination based on case reports. Thirty-two percent of male Connecticut survivors said they were rejected from employment compared to 21 percent of the controls. The reported female survivor and sibling rejection experiences, on the other hand, were very similar. Based on the Connecticut data, a history of a childhood or adolescent malignancy appears to be a greater impediment to males in the workplace than to females. This may reflect the higher levels of occupational opportunities and training to which men aspire and which men are often offered. The examination of job category and income level for males vs. females using data from the NCI questionnaire support this. The sex-related patterns of rejection may unfortunately become more similar as increased numbers of women pursue higher education and professional status.

These data provide supporting evidence that insurance companies tend to reject childhood and adolescent cancer survivors and are consistent with published reports related to cancer patients in general (Fitzgerald 1981; Modjeska 1977). Our control group's ability to obtain life insurance was remarkably similar to that of the U.S. population. A 1972 survey found that 97 percent of life insurance applicants were successful (Fitzgerald 1981). This rate is identical to that of the male sibling population and 2 percent lower than the female siblings. The Mayo Comprehensive Cancer Center's 1976 survey of insurance underwriting practices reported differentiation with respect to tumor type, a factor not found to be associated with denials in this investigation (Mayo Study 1977). This may be attributable to changes in insurance practice over the 30-year period of observation of the present investigation; or the fact that insurance companies weigh a variety of factors in addition to type of cancer, such as time since diagnosis, in their decisions.

Insurance carriers have readily discussed their standards for cancer survivors (Fitzgerald 1981; Modjeska 1977; Mayo Study 1977). Employers have been generally silent regarding hiring policies. An exception is the Metropolitan Life Insurance Company, which selectively employed persons with a history of cancer and conducted a prospective survey of their health and service record (Cunnick, et al. 1974). Their reported employment acceptance rate for cancer history patients was 50 percent, depending on whether there was "a reasonable expectation of continuous service." These individuals were found to have a good health record after employment and reasonably low absenteeism.

It is unknown how often insurance companies and potential employers approached by study subjects from the present investigation were aware of the applicants' medical histories. One man, diagnosed as a child with Wilm's tumor, reported completing three hundred job applications without receiving a single response. He claimed to have been honest in declaring all his hospitalizations on the applications. Another man had difficulty obtaining a position even after his physician intervened. Complaints to the state labor board also did not help. Another reported being rejected after a potential employer reviewed his medical record and discovered that he had a serious spine abnormality. One woman was advised by her doctor to say she had polio as a child, rather than cancer when applying for jobs. Some cases reported that they denied having been diagnosed with cancer when applying for insurance (and employment) or failed to ever apply for fear of rejection. The special problems of those left physically handicapped because of their disease experiences in childhood are striking. They constitute a subgroup of the survivor population at high risk for denial of both employment and insurance. One woman denied a job said, "I was asked how I would be able to walk to serve coffee with crutches." Vision problems presented employment and insurance difficulties for several survivors. Plastic surgery to correct visible X-ray burns on one man's face considerably improved his job prospects.

Of the survivors, 30 percent were ignorant of their childhood malignancy themselves at the time of the interview and could, therefore, not have informed institutions to which they were making an application for employment or insurance. Almost all survivor respondents were cognizant, however, of a hospitalization as a child. The "true" frequency of denials due to diagnosis of childhood or adolescent cancer may in fact be greater than respondents perceive them to be.

It should be noted that these results were based on the numbers who themselves applied for insurance and did not include those who received insurance automatically through their own employment or that of their spouses. For long-term survivors of childhood cancer, employability takes on added importance as an avenue to obtaining health and life insurance.

The length of the main NCI questionnaire constrained the amount of data which could be collected in the Connecticut Addendum; consequently, it lacked in-depth information. The findings derived from the data on realization of major socioeconomic goals must therefore be interpreted cautiously. There are no independent sources of data to confirm the reported denials or to verify whether the reasons for rejection are consistent with respondent perceptions. The variation in percentages providing affirmative answers for the different goals examined and the similarity of survivor and sibling female responses to job denials give reasonable assurance that survivors did not bias the results. Sibling comparisons preclude factors related to genetic or socioeconomic background from explaining the differences observed.

For all socioeconomic objectives the respondents were asked if they were "ever denied." These findings, therefore, do not necessarily reflect permanent rejection or current status. An independent addendum to the NCI questionnaire, administered in Kansas, addressed the percentages of study subjects with insurance in force at the time of interview (Holmes, et al. 1986). Survivors in the Kansas cohort were found to be significantly less likely than their siblings to have life or health insurance coverage. It is also of interest that both studies report the rate for life insurance problems to be twice as high as that for health insurance. The absolute frequencies from the Connecticut and Kansas addenda, although specific to the same diagnostic time period, cannot be directly compared due to difference in addenda questionnaire designs. The overall conclusions, however, are the same.

CONCLUSIONS

This investigation examined the socioeconomic effects of extended survival of childhood and adolescent cancer. On the encouraging side there is supportable evidence that long-term survivors, with the exception of those diagnosed with brain tumors, achieve educational goals comparable to their siblings. Despite the attainment of academic parity, however, survivors experience poorer occupational performance and report a higher frequency of employment rejections. Both male and female survivors report significantly more difficulty obtaining health and life insurance than do their brothers and sisters. Legislative initiatives as well as awareness programs for insurance providers and potential employers are clearly needed to ameliorate the employment and insurability problems for current and future cancer survivors of all ages.

REFERENCES

Cunnick, W. R., Cromie, J. B., Cortell, R. E., & Wright, B. P. Employing the cancer patient: A mutual responsibility. *Journal of Occupational Medicine*, 1974, *16*, 775–780.

Duffner, P. K., Cohen, M. D., Patrick, R. M., et al. The long-term effects of cranial irradiation on the central nervous system. *Cancer*, 1985, *56*, 1841–1846.

Endicott, J., & Spitzer, R. L. A diagnostic interview: The schedule for affective disorders and schizophrenia. *Archives of General Psychiatry*, 1978, *35*, 837–844.

Fitzgerald, R. H. Life insurance after malignant disease. *Annals of Internal Medicine*, 1981, *95*, 633–635.

Holmes, G. E., Baker, A., Hassanein, R. S., Bovee, E. C., Mulvihill, J. J., Myers, M. H., & Holmes, F. F. The availability of insurance to long-time survivors of childhood cancer. *Cancer*, 1986, *57*, 190–193.

Holmes, H. A., & Holmes, F. F. After ten years, what are the handicaps and life styles of children treated for cancer? *Clinical Pediatrics*, 1975, *14*, 819–823.

Koocher, G. P., & O'Malley, J. E. *The Damocles syndrome: Psychosocial consequences of surviving childhood cancer.* New York: McGraw-Hill, 1981.

Li, F. P., & Stone, R. Survivors of cancer in childhood. *Annals of Internal Medicine*, 1976, *84*, 551–553.

Mayo Comprehensive Cancer Center. *A study of discrimination toward cancer patients by insurers, employers and vocational rehabilitation agencies.* Rochester, MI: Mayo Clinic, 1977, p. 103.

Meadows, A. T., & Sibler, J. Delayed consequences of therapy for childhood cancer. *CA—A Cancer Journal for Clinicians*, 1985, *35*, 271–286.

Modjeska, G. S. Insurance and the cancer patient. In *Proceedings of the American Cancer Society second national conference on human values and cancer.* New York: American Cancer Society, 1977, 198–203.

Schiefelbein, S. *Surviving childhood cancer.* New York: Memorial Sloan Kettering Cancer Center, 1981.

Spitzer, R. L., Endicott, J., & Robins, E. Research diagnostic criteria. *Archives of General Psychiatry*, 1978, *35*, 773–782.

Teta, M. J., Del Po, M. A., Kasl, S. V., Meigs, J. W., Myers, M. H., & Mulvihill, J. J. Psychosocial consequences of childhood and adolescent cancer survival. *Journal of Chronic Diseases*, 1986, *39*, 751–759.

4

Insurance Experiences of Childhood Cancer Survivors

Grace E. Holmes, Ariel B. Baker, Frederick F. Holmes, and Ruth S. Hassanein

INTRODUCTION

In the past, for many, a diagnosis of cancer meant an inevitable and relatively rapid death. However, with the advent of new and combined treatment regimens, beginning in the 1960s, survival rates from cancer have improved greatly. It is estimated that of over 5 million Americans alive today in the mid–1980s with a history of cancer, at least 60 percent have survived more than five years (McKenna 1984). Further, a majority of these over 3 million survivors are considered cured of cancer.

Among those who make up these encouraging figures are long-term survivors of childhood cancer. Today, the survival rate of children diagnosed with cancer has increased substantially (Boren, et al. 1985; D'Angio 1977; Feldman, et al. 1980; Hartman, et al. 1977; Holmes & Holmes 1975; Koocher & O'Malley 1981) and their overall survival rate now exceeds 50 percent. One study estimates that by the year 1990, one in 1000 individuals reaching age 20 will be a cured survivor of both childhood cancer and its therapy (Feldman, et al. 1980).

Children with cancer can now be given the hope and opportunity to realize a normal life span (Hartman, et al. 1977). These survivors can look back on many hurdles they have overcome. They and their families have confronted numerous emotional, psychological, and financial crises, in addition to the physical suffering of the cancer as well as the treatment.

As these young cancer survivors reach adulthood, attempt to enter the job force, and begin productive adult lives, they encounter new difficulties that appear in the form of discrimination because of their prior cancer history (Feldman, et al. 1980; Mayo Clinic Study 1977). One form of discrimination experienced by long-term childhood cancer survivors has occurred with attempts to obtain life and health insurance (Feldman, et al. 1980; Koocher & O'Malley 1981).

Insurance has become a major institution in our nation (Modjeska 1977). It is estimated that 90 percent of Americans have health coverage and over 150 million Americans hold life insurance worth more than $2.1 trillion (Fitzgerald 1981; McKenna 1984; Modjeska 1977). To many people, insurance coverage symbolizes independence, security, and success.

Although some insurance companies already acknowledge that individuals treated for childhood cancer will have a normal life span (Ashenberg 1975), refusals, restricted policies, and higher premiums for these people still occur (Feldman, et al. 1980; Koocher & O'Malley 1981; Mayo Study 1977; McKenna 1984). Some persons who have survived childhood cancer anticipate this situation and may be reluctant to apply for insurance, even after many years have elapsed from time of diagnosis and treatment (Modjeska 1977).

Actuarial survival data for long-term survivors of childhood cancer are not available. Those tables that are used to determine degree of risk, lag somewhat behind more current prognoses and do not necessarily reflect future survival rates (Ashenberg 1975; Fitzgerald 1981; McKenna 1985).

In early 1981 a five-institution collaborative study was conducted on the long-term morbidity and mortality of adults who survived childhood cancer and their siblings (Mulvihill et al. 1984). The purpose was to obtain data regarding the current health of the cases and their sibling controls as well as achievement in education and the work force, occurrence of second cancers, outcome of pregnancies, and the health of their offspring.

Five institutions—the University of Kansas, the University of Iowa, the University of Texas, Yale University, and the California State Department of Health Services—collaborated in this effort to study the fates of over 2200 long-term childhood cancer survivors and 3000 of their siblings.

The University of Kansas Medical Center obtained additional information about life and health insurance from their cases and control siblings (Holmes, et al. 1986). This was done in order to compare the ease or difficulty in obtaining insurance coverage as well as the amount of coverage in both cases and controls.

Subjects and Methods

Since its inception in 1945, the Tumor Registry of the University of Kansas Medical Center (KUMC) has maintained a 99.9 percent follow-up rate of cancer patients. To date, of the 42,258 cancer patients registered, only 24 have been lost to follow-up.

In 1981 at the onset of the five-institution collaborative study of long-term morbidity and mortality of adults who survived childhood cancer, the whereabouts of all childhood cancer survivors was known. In order to qualify for the study, subjects must have survived at least five years after diagnosis and must have reached the age of 21 years by December 31, 1979. Some cases were deceased but had met all criteria.

There were 268 persons who fit the above criteria and who were diagnosed and treated for cancer between birth and 19 years of age during the period between 1945 and 1974. Siblings of these cases served as controls.

Two control siblings per case were chosen whenever possible. Their participation was based on the factors of blood relationship, sex, and age, in that order, matched to the case sibling. In some instances, there were no controls or only one.

Interviews of cases and controls were conducted using a pre-tested questionnaire which covered education, occupation, tobacco and drug use, marital status, general health, reproductive history, and health status of children.

An addendum to the questionnaire for Kansas cases and controls included four questions about health and life insurance. These were: (1) Have you ever experienced difficulty getting life insurance because of reasons of health? (2) How many dollars in life insurance of all kinds do you have in force now? (3) Have you ever had difficulty in obtaining health insurance because of health reasons? and (4) Do you have health insurance coverage now? The wording was appropriately modified for interview of a proxy when necessary. Trained interviewers were able to administer the entire questionnaire and addendum in approximately one hour.

Cases were contacted initially with a letter introducing the research project and noting that they were members of a select group of people who had survived a serious childhood illness. For those who were deceased, a letter, appropriately modified, was sent to a close relative to arrange for an interview.

Controls were selected and contacted after names of siblings, addresses, and telephone numbers were obtained from cases. Occasionally, a case advised interviewers that a sibling might wish not to be interviewed. Such requests were honored by interviewers.

Cases and controls were interviewed in person whenever possible and some interviews were conducted by telephone. When a case or control was deceased, incompetent, or unavailable, a family member was interviewed as proxy.

Data were analyzed using chi-square test and the phi coefficient to show relationship between two variables for all cases and all controls, for male cases versus controls, for female cases versus controls, and in some instances, for males versus females within the case and control groups. In addition, McNemar's statistical test for the significance of changes was used with data from a large sub-group of one hundred tightly matched case/same-sex control pairs, reported on previously (Mulvihill et al. 1984).

Results

Of the 268 cases who fulfilled the study criteria, interviews, which included the questions regarding insurance, were conducted with 264 cases and 369 controls or their proxies. From this number, however, one was under 21 years of age, 38 cases were dead, six cases had no controls, three had not been asked the questions regarding insurance, and two were incompetent at the time of the interview, leaving a total of 214 cases and their 302 controls.

A comparison of the case and control groups and sex subgroups with regard to the factors of age at time of interview, attained educational level, and marital status are shown in Table 4.1. Mean age for cases and controls was identical, 33.9 years. No significant differences were found between the groups or gender subgroups in regard to highest grade completed, percentage of high school graduates, or percentage of those completing 16 years or more of school. A larger percentage of female cases versus controls attained higher educational levels, approaching significance. In addition, there was a significantly larger number of control males (33.3%) versus females (17.1%) with higher educational attainment, $p < 0.01$.

Marital information showed no significant differences between cases and controls with regard to being married at the time of the interview, never having married, or being divorced at the time of the interview. Among the cases more females (71.6%) than males (53.6%) were married, $p < 0.01$, and more male (29.5%) than female (12.7%) cases had never married, $p < 0.01$. No significant differences were seen between male and female controls.

Table 4.2 compares employment histories and current income of cases and controls. There were seven cases and six controls who had never been employed, a nonsignificant difference. However, among controls, all six were women, showing a significant sex difference, $p < 0.05$. Some of the never employed were homemakers who had not sought out-of-home employment.

Interviewees were asked to name the type of job in which they were employed the longest over their adult work life. Categories from which to choose were: farming, skilled labor, unskilled labor, professional (health field), professional (other), clerical, managerial, never employed, and don't know.

The three leading types of employment for males, both cases and controls, were skilled labor (cases = 32.1%, controls = 32.6%), professional health field and other (cases = 27.7%, controls = 27.8%), and unskilled labor (cases = 16.1%, controls = 13.2%). For females, professional work (health field and other) was most common (cases = 34.3%, controls = 27.8%), followed by clerical (cases = 32.4%, controls = 25.9%). The third leading type of employment for female cases was skilled labor (12.7%) and for female controls, unskilled labor (19.0%).

More cases missed work because of health reasons than did controls, p < 0.001 for all, p < 0.01 for males, p < 0.001 for females. Mean annual income of all cases and gender subgroups was just about the same as their controls.

Not all of our cases and controls were able to provide us with insurance information. However, responses to the questions regarding difficulty in obtaining health or life insurance because of health reasons indicated that of 208 cases for whom this information was available, 41 (19.7%) had difficulty in obtaining health insurance compared to only five of 299 controls (1.7%), p < 0.001. This same significant difference applied to gender subgroups (see Table 4.3).

Likewise, with life insurance, 91 of 205 cases (44.4%) had difficulty getting life insurance whereas only 13 of 302 controls (4.3%) had such difficulty, p < 0.001. This significant difference was also present when comparing cases and controls according to sex (see Table 4.4).

When interviewees were asked if they owned either health or life insurance, 180 of 213 cases (84.5%) and 262 of 298 controls (87.9%) had health insurance, demonstrating no significant difference between the groups and subgroups (see Table 4.5). However, only 123 of 192 cases (64.1%) were owners of life insurance compared to 210 of 255 controls (82.4%), p < 0.001 (for males, p < 0.01, females p < 0.002) (see Table 4.6). In addition, a significant difference between sexes existed for both cases (p < 0.05) and controls (p < 0.01) due to smaller percentages of women who owned life insurance.

Table 4.7 shows mean life insurance ownership amounts by all cases versus all controls as well as for the gender subgroups. Mean amounts of life insurance are much less for all cases ($26,045) than for all controls ($39,386) and according to gender comparison. Further, females of both groups have the smallest amounts of coverage.

Median amounts of life insurance ownership for all groups and subgroups are shown in Table 4.8. Because of lack of ownership by 69 cases and 45 controls, median amounts are low and more dramatically reflect the above differences between the various groups.

When data of 100 case/same-sex controls were compared using them as pairs or dyads and applying McNemar's analysis, the childhood cancer survivors had significantly more difficulty obtaining health insurance because of health reasons than their same-sex sibling controls (p < 0.001) (see Table 4.9), and were less likely than controls to be covered by health insurance (p < 0.04) (see Table 4.10). Female cases and controls, however,

Table 4.1
Comparison of Cases and Controls (Age, Education, Marital Status)

		Cases			Controls		
1. Mean age (years)							
	All	*n=214	33.9	(25-55)	n=302	33.9	(22-59)	NS**
	Male	n=112	33.1	(25-55)	n=144	34.0	(22-59)	NS
	Female	n=102	34.8	(25-52)	n=158	33.8	(22-53)	NS
2. Median age (years)							
	All	n=214	34.0		n=302	33.0		NS
3. Education (Highest grade completed)							
	All	n=214	13.3	(2-19)	n=302	13.5	(8-19)	NS
	Male	n=112	13.1	(2-19)	n=144	14.0	(8-19)	NS
	Female	n=102	13.5	(6-19)	n=158	13.1	(9-19)	NS
4. High School graduates (number)							
	All	n=214	188	(87. 9%)	n=302	272	(90.1%)	NS
	Male	n=112	94	(83. 9%)	n=144	129	(89.6%)	NS
	Female	n=102	94	(92. 2%)	n=158	143	(90.5%)	NS
5. Completion of - 16 years of school (number)							
	All	n=214	55	(25. 7%)	n=302	75	(24.8%)	NS
	Male	n=112	28	(25. 0%)	n=144	48	(33.3%)	NS
	Female	n=102	27	(26. 5%)	n=158	27	(17.1%)	NS

6. Marital data:

Presently married (number)

	Case			Controls			p-value
All	n=214	133	(62.1%)	n=302	194	(64.2%)	NS
Male	n=112	60	(53.6%)	n=144	91	(63.2%)	NS
Female	n=102	73	(71.6%)	n=158	103	(65.2%)	NS

Never married (number)

	Case			Controls			p-value
All	n=214	46	(21.5%)	n=302	51	(16.9%)	NS
Male	n=112	33	(29.5%)	n=144	28	(19.4%)	NS
Female	n=102	13	(12.7%)	n=158	23	(14.6%)	NS

Divorced (number)

	Case			Controls			p-value
All	n=214	25	(11.7%)	n=302	33	(10.9%)	NS
Male	n=112	10	(8.9%)	n=144	15	(10.4%)	NS
Female	n=102	15	(14.7%)	n=158	18	(11.4%)	NS

*n=number

**NS=not significant

Source: Compiled by the authors.

Table 4.2
Comparison of Cases and Controls (Employment and Income)

		Cases		Controls		p-value
1. Never employed (number)						
All	n=214	7	(3.3%)	n=302	6	(2.0%)	NS
Male	n=112	2	(1.8%)	n=144	0	(0.0%)	NS
Female	n=102	5	(4.9%)	n=158	6	(3.8%)	NS
2. Missed more than 3 months work because of health reasons						
All	n=214	60	(24.0%)	n=302	30	(9.9%)	NS
Male	n=112	32	(28.6%)	n=144	18	(12.5%)	NS
Female	n=102	28	(27.5%)	n=158	12	(7.6%)	NS
3. Mean annual income						
All	n=204	$16,691	($10,000-60,000)	n=291	$17,182	($10,000-60,000)	
Male	n=108	$20,532	($10,000-60,000)	n=140	$21,571	($10,000-60,000)	
Female	n=96	$12,369	($10,000-60,000)	n=151	$13,112	($10,000-37,500)	

Source: Compiled by authors.

Table 4.3
Report of Difficulty Obtaining Health Insurance

	Cases			Controls			p-value
All	n=208	41	(19.7%)	n=299	5	(1.7%)	< 0.001
Male	n=107	21	(19.6%)	n=142	1	(0.7%)	< 0.001
Female	n=101	20	(19.8%)	n=157	4	(2.5%)	< 0.001

Source: Compiled by the authors.

Table 4.4
Report of Difficulty Obtaining Life Insurance

	Cases			Controls			p-value
All	n=205	91	(44.4%)	n=302	13	(4.3%)	< 0.001
Male	n=107	47	(43.9%)	n=144	5	(3.5%)	< 0.001
Female	n= 98	44	(44.9%)	n=158	8	(5.1%)	< 0.001

Source: Compiled by the authors.

Table 4.5
Own Health Insurance

	Cases			Controls			p-value
All	n=213	180	(84.5%)	n=298	262	(87.9%)	NS
Male	n=112	94	(83.9%)	n=142	127	(89.4%)	NS
Female	n=101	86	(85.1%)	n=156	135	(86.5%)	NS

Source: Compiled by the authors.

Table 4.6
Own Life Insurance

	Cases			Controls			p-value
All	n=192	123	(64.1%)	n=255	210	(82.4%)	< 0.001
Male	n=100	72	(72.0%)	n=128	114	(89.1%)	< 0.01
Female	n= 92	51	(55.4%)	n=127	96	(75.6%)	< 0.002

Source: Compiled by the authors.

Table 4.7
Life Insurance Ownership, Mean Amounts

	Cases			Controls		
All	n=192	$26,045	($0-350,000)	n=255	$39,386	($0-500,000)
Male	n=100	$40,317	($0-350,000)	n=128	$59,746	($0-500,0C0)
Female	n= 92	$10,533	($0-215,000)	n=127	$18,866	($0-250,000)

Source: Compiled by authors.

Table 4.8
Life Insurance Ownership, Median Amounts

		Cases		Controls
All	n=123	$ 8,000	n=210	$15,000
Male	n= 72	$16,000	n=114	$30,000
Female	n= 51	$ 2,000	n= 96	$ 8,000

Source: Compiled by the authors.

Table 4.9
Report of Difficulty Obtaining Health Insurance (100 Case/Same-Sex Siblings)

		Cases	Controls	p-value
All	n=100	24 (24.0%)	0 (0%)	< 0.001
Male	n= 58	13 (22.4%)	0 (0%)	< 0.001
Female	n= 42	11 (26.2%)	0 (0%)	< 0.001

Source: Compiled by the authors.

Table 4.10
Own Health Insurance (100 Case/Same-Sex Siblings)

		Cases	Controls	p-value
All	n=99	84 (84.8%)	92 (92.9%)	0.04
Male	n=58	50 (86.2%)	56 (96.6%)	0.04
Female	n=41	34 (82.9%)	36 (87.8%)	NS

Source: Compiled by the authors.

Table 4.11
Report of Difficulty Obtaining Life Insurance (100 Cases/Same-Sex Siblings)

		Cases	Controls	p-value
All	n=98	44 (44.9%)	2 (2.0%)	< 0.001
Male	n=58	25 (43.1%)	2 (3.4%)	< 0.001
Female	n=40	19 (47.5%)	0 (0.0%)	< 0.001

Source; Compiled by the authors.

were not significantly different in the coverage of health insurance (Holmes, et al. 1986).

Applying the same analysis, childhood cancer survivors had more difficulty obtaining life insurance than their controls (p < 0.001) (see Table 4.11), they were much less likely to have life insurance in force (p < 0.004) (see Table 4.12), and had smaller amounts of life insurance dollars in force (see Table 4.13). When determining median amounts for only those with life insurance from among the one hundred pairs, all cases have less than

Table 4.12
Own Life Insurance (100 Case/Same-Sex Siblings)

		Cases		Controls		p-value
All	n=100	70	(70.0%)	87	(87.0%)	<0.004
Male	n= 58	46	(79.3%)	54	(93.1%)	<0.04
Female	n= 42	24	(57.1%)	33	(78.6%)	<0.04

Source: Compiled by the authors.

Table 4.13
Median Amounts of Life Insurance Dollars in Force (100 Cases/Same-Sex Siblings)

		Cases	Controls
All	n=100	$12,000	$22,000
Male	n= 58	$25,000	$45,000
Female	n= 42	$ 4,000	$10,000

Source: Compiled by the authors.

Table 4.14
Median Amounts of Life Insurance in Force of Those Having Insurance (100 Cases/Same-Sex Siblings)

	Cases		Controls	
All	n=70	$24,000	n=87	$28,000
Male	n=46	$36,000	n=54	$48,000
Female	n=24	$10,000	n=33	$10,000

Source: Compiled by the authors.

controls except for female cases versus female controls (see Table 4.14) (Holmes, et al. 1986).

Discussion

Recent data from this institution have shown that childhood cancer survivors are at significant disadvantage in our society with regard to obtaining both life and health insurance. The one hundred pairs of tightly matched case/same-sex sibling controls reported on by Holmes, et al. (1986) demonstrated much less likelihood of ownership of life insurance by cases versus controls. Differences in health insurance ownership, though less marked, were still present (see Tables 4.9–4.12).

Expansion of data analysis included and compared all available cases and controls in addition to the one hundred pairs reported above. The results of the larger groups of 214 cases and 302 controls reflected in general the reported results of the one hundred case/control pairs.

In comparing the large groups of cases and controls in Tables 4.1 and 4.2, there is little difference in mean values with regard to most factors. The mean age of each group was 33.9 years, cases ranged from 25 to 55 years, and controls from 22 to 59 years. Age differed slightly in gender subgroups but was not significant. Median age for the two groups also was not significantly different (cases = 34 years, controls = 33 years). Thus, most of these people should have been quite well settled in life.

The educational level completed was similar for cases (13.3 years) and controls (13.5 years). The range of educational levels indicates that some cases completed only a few years of schooling. There was one male case with a second grade education, one male and one female case with sixth grade educations and one male case with a seventh grade education. This was offset, however, among the cases by many high attainers of education. None of the controls had less than eight years of formal education.

The data show that female cases tended to have a higher mean educational level than did either the female controls or the male cases. Further, the female cases had a higher percentage of high school graduates than the male cases and both control groups. They also had a higher percentage (26.5%) completing 16 or more years of schooling than the male cases (25%) and remarkably higher than the female controls (17.1%), but not higher than the male controls (33.3%). This suggests they are a group of determined achievers.

The marital picture was not significantly different between all cases and controls. However, female cases were more likely than male cases to have been married at the time of the interview, while male cases were more likely never to have married.

The factor of never having been employed was not striking for either group nor significantly different. Highly significant, however, was the factor of ever missing more than three months of work because of health reasons, being more likely among the cases than the controls, which one might expect.

The employment picture shows a similar pattern of mostly skilled labor, professional work, and unskilled labor among male cases accounting for 75.9 percent and controls accounting for 73.6 percent. However, professional fields ranked first among the women, followed by clerical work, then by skilled labor for female cases and unskilled labor for female controls. Those categories accounted for 79.4 percent of female cases and 72.7 percent of female controls. It appears that employment sought by female cases reflects a similar determination as did their education picture.

Mean annual income is lower among controls but not significantly so. The large discrepancy is sex related and reflects the currently accepted data that women generally receive approximately 60 percent as much income as men even when similarly employed (Holden 1986; Wright 1982).

In the area of reported difficulty in obtaining health or life insurance because of health reasons, 19.7 percent of all cases had difficulty obtaining health insurance compared to only 1.7 percent of all controls, thus more than ten times more likely to have had problems. A similar trend existed for gender subgroups (see Table 4.3).

Life insurance was even more difficult for cases to obtain: 44.4 percent of all cases versus 4.3 percent of all controls had a problem in this area, again being about ten times more difficult (see Table 4.4). With both health and life insurance, female cases had the most difficulty and male controls the least in obtaining insurance.

When asked, however, if they currently had health insurance coverage (see Table 4.5), there was no significant difference between all cases (84.5%) and all controls (87.9%). The least difference noted was between female cases and female controls. On the other hand, life insurance ownership (see Table 4.6), showed significant differences between all cases (64.1%) and all controls (82.4%) as well as the gender subgroups. Again, female cases were least likely to own life insurance (55.4%) and male controls were most likely (89.1%). For those who owned life insurance the dollar amount was highest among male controls and lowest among female cases (see Tables 4.7 and 4.8).

The insurance picture from the published data of the one hundred cases/ same-sex sibling controls was very similar to the results from the larger group (Tables 4.9–4.12). One exception was the lack of significant difference between all cases and controls in the larger group in the ownership of health insurance (Table 4.5 versus Table 4.11). It is not known how many women, either cases or controls, may have had health insurance coverage through their husband's employment, regardless of their own health histories. There were 85.1 percent of all female cases and 86.5 percent of all female controls who had health insurance coverage, whereas 83.9 percent of all male cases had health insurance compared to 89.4 percent of all male controls.

These data provide ample evidence that childhood cancer survivors, both male and female, are likely to be deprived of an opportunity to obtain life and health insurance with the same ease as their siblings. Utilizing both total data as well as the large subgroup of one hundred cases and controls, only 0–2.5 percent of controls experienced difficulty obtaining health insurance yet about 20–25 percent of childhood cancer survivors had difficulty. Life insurance was even more difficult for survivors to obtain, approaching 50 percent as opposed to 0–5 percent for controls.

In spite of this difficulty the childhood cancer survivors do own health insurance, in almost the same percentage as their controls. This is the only bright spot in the insurance experience picture. It is not known how many of our survivors with health insurance concealed their past cancer diagnosis in order to obtain insurance.

Childhood cancer survivors also do own life insurance but in significantly fewer numbers than the control group and have significantly smaller amounts of dollar ownership. The cases should be commended for pursuing their right to these benefits in the face of resistance by our society and by insurance companies.

It is ironic that the group noted to have achieved such high educational levels, namely the female cases, should be apparently penalized with regard to life insurance acquisition and should also have the smallest amounts of life insurance ownership. In this regard, one must also consider that amounts of life insurance coverage are, in part, a result of personal choice.

Persons cured of childhood cancer can make plans for their adult lives. Besides education, employment, and marriage, a natural part of their plans will include health and life insurance coverage. As more survival data become available to insurance companies, realistic flexibility should be seriously considered by and expected from these companies. Survivors, their families, and society in general demand that childhood cancer survivors be allowed access to the same rights and privileges that their siblings and peers already enjoy. A great deal of ingenuity, imagination, and cooperation will be required by all who have chosen to help in the solution to this complex problem.

CONCLUSION

Childhood cancer survivors, now adults (n = 214), and their siblings (n = 302) were interviewed about their health, education, employment, marital status, health of offspring, and, in addition, were asked about their experiences in obtaining and owning life and health insurance. The cases and controls were similar in age (33.9 years) and highest grade completed (13.3 and 13.5 years) though a higher percentage of female cases were high school graduates (NS). Male controls were more likely to have had 16 years or more of schooling followed by the female cases. Marital status at the time of interview was similar for cases and controls.

Cases were significantly more likely than controls to have missed more than three months of work because of health reasons. Common types of employment of cases and controls are discussed as well as mean income.

There was a significant difference (p < 0.001) between cases and controls in the difficulty encountered by cases in obtaining both health and life insurance. In spite of this, many cases had health insurance and, though in fewer numbers than controls, this was not significant. Many cases also owned life insurance, but in significantly fewer numbers than controls (p < 0.001) and smaller amounts.

Childhood cancer survivors deserve the same opportunity to obtain insurance coverage as their siblings without a history of cancer. Updated actuarial tables for use by insurance companies are clearly needed to address this important social and human rights issue. Special advocacy and counseling services for survivors may help to minimize or even eliminate the reported difficulties.

REFERENCES

Ashenberg, N.J. Employability and insurability of the cancer patient. Paper presented at the New York State Cancer Programs Association, Inc. Rochester, NY: November 8, 1975.

Boren, H., Adams, P., & Ried, H. Educational levels and occupations of long-term survivors of childhood cancers. In *Tenth annual mental health conference. Childhood cancer survivors: Living beyond cure.* Houston: The University of Texas, M. D. Anderson Hospital and Tumor Institute at Houston, 1985, 3.

D'Angio, G.J. Late adversities of treatment of long-term survivors of childhood cancer. In *Proceedings of the American Cancer Society second national conference of human values and cancer.* New York: American Cancer Society, 1977, 59.

Feldman, F.L. *Work and cancer health histories: Work expectations and experiences of youth with cancer histories (ages 13–23).* Oakland, CA: American Cancer Society, California Division, 1980.

Fitzgerald, R.H. Life insurance after malignant diseases. *Annals of Internal Medicine,* 1981, *95,* 633–635.

Hartman, J.R., Rudolph, L. A., Trull, P., Johnson, F. L., & Hutchinson, F. Cancer—The child and the adolescent—Part I. Introduction. In *Proceedings of the American Cancer Society second national conference of human values and cancer.* New York: American Cancer Society, 1977, 15–18.

Holden, C. Working women still segregated and underpaid. *Science,* 1986, *231,* 449.

Holmes, G. E., Baker, A., Hassanein, R. S., Bovee, E. C., Mulvihill, J. J., Myers, M. H., & Holmes, F. F. The availability of insurance to long-term survivors of childhood cancer. *Cancer,* 1986, *57,* 190–193.

Holmes, H. A. & Holmes, F. F. After ten years, what are the handicaps and life styles of children treated for cancer? *Clinical Pediatrics,* 1975, *14,* 819–823.

Koocher, G. P., and O'Malley, J. E. *The Damocles syndrome: Psychosocial consequences of surviving childhood cancer.* New York: McGraw-Hill, 1981, 122–124.

Mayo Comprehensive Cancer Center. A study of discrimination toward cancer patients by insurers, employees and vocational rehabilitation agencies. Rochester, MI: Mayo Clinic, 1977.

McKenna, R J. Employment and insurance issues for the cancer patient. In *Proceedings of the fourth national conference on cancer nursing—1983.* New York: American Cancer Society, Inc., 1984, 36–46.

McKenna, R. J. We could save more lives. *Cancer News, an American Cancer Society, Inc. Publication,* 1985, Winter, 1.

Modjeska, G. S. Insurance and the cancer patient. In *Proceedings of the American Cancer Society second national conference on human values and cancer.* New York: American Cancer Society, 1977, 198–203.

Mulvihill, J. J., Myers, M. H., Steinhorn, S. C., et al. Cancer in offspring of long-time survivors of childhood and adolescent cancer. *Lancet,* 1987, 2: 813–817.

Wright, J. C. *The American almanac of jobs and salaries.* New York: Avon Books, 1982, 745–746.

5

Illness and Nonillness Causes of Work-related Problems Among Persons with Cancer

Peter S. Houts, S. Benham Kahn, Joyce M. Yasco, Joan F. Hermann, Allan Lipton, George W. Schelzel, Katherine M. Marconi, and Mary J. Bartholomew

An important and, up to now, unanswered question about employment problems experienced by persons with cancer (PWC) is the degree to which cancer alone causes employment problems and to what degree noncancer problems also contribute. This question is important because, in order to be effective in helping PWC with these problems, it is necessary to understand their causes. For example, different strategies are called for when persons with cancer experience problems that grow out of a long history of employer-employee conflict than when problems occur only in the context of having cancer. Both types of employment problems should be addressed since they both could affect a PWC's ability to cope with the disease. However, the interventions that will be effective are likely to be different when the problems result from different causes. By comparing the problem-reporting rates of persons with and without cancer, we can estimate the degree to which cancer, alone, caused people to report problems and the degree to which problems reported by PWC involved other causes as well. The rate at which persons without cancer report problems can be taken as the "baseline problem rate." Differences between PWCs' rates and these baseline rates are an indication of how cancer changes problem reporting. The overlap in their reporting rates is an indication of the extent to which PWCs' problems involve causes in addition to the cancer, though the cancer may still affect how those problems are expressed.

Another important kind of information that has been missing is population estimates of the percent and numbers of persons with cancer who experience work-related problems. This is important information for organizing programs on a state or national basis to deal with these needs. Earlier studies have suggested that work-related problems may be common among employed persons with cancer (Feldman 1976, 1978; Greenleigh Associates 1979; Mellete 1985). Problems reported include lack of promotions, exclusion from health insurance or other benefits, and problems in PWCs' relations with fellow workers and supervisors. However, the different studies have selected samples in different ways, each with its own potential sources of bias and none have attempted to correct for these biases to make estimates for a state or the nation as a whole.

In this chapter we present data which address both of these issues. First, we estimate the frequency with which employed PWC report job-related problems in a large and culturally diverse geographical area, namely the state of Pennsylvania. Second, we will estimate the degree to which employed PWC would experience similar employment problems even without a diagnosis of cancer by comparing the employment problems reported by employed PWC with those reported by their employed same-sex siblings without cancer for the same time periods. To provide further insight into the causes of PWC employment problems, we have also examined the characteristics of PWC most likely to report employment-related problems following their diagnoses. It should be noted that this study was concerned only with problems experienced by employed PWC and did not address problems PWC may have in obtaining new employment.

HOW THE DATA WERE OBTAINED

The findings presented here are part of a larger study of the problems experienced by cancer patients conducted for the Pennsylvania Department of Health. The methods used to obtain these data are explained in detail elsewhere (Houts, et al. 1986). We briefly summarize those aspects of the methodology that are important for understanding the findings presented here. Participants in this study were selected from the Pennsylvania Cancer Registry. Approximately equal numbers of respondents were selected from three age groups: 20–39, 40–64, and >64 years of age. Nonmalignant skin cancers and in situ cervical cancers were excluded from the sample because the excellent prognosis and limited treatments required by those groups would minimize the impact of cancer on their lives. A total of 629 interviews were conducted.

Respondents were asked about a wide range of problems that could have occurred since the PWCs' diagnoses. Included were five questions concerning employment. Responses to these five questions are the subject of this chapter. These questions were asked only of those PWCs who were employed at some time since their diagnoses. The questions dealt with problems in doing the job; problems with supervisors or co-workers, with the amount of money the respondent was able to earn, with insurance benefits provided by the employer; and problems in keeping the job. PWCs were first asked if they had experienced these problems at any time since the date of their diagnoses. If they answered yes, they were asked if it was "very much," "some," or a "little" problem. Scoring of responses to the job-related problem questions was dichotomous. Responses of "very much" or "some" were scored indicating a problem while responses of "little" or "no" were scored as no problem.

A sample of same-sex siblings of PWC were identified in the following manner. Interviews with PWC were conducted in random order and the first PWCs interviewed were asked if they had a live same-sex sibling. If the respondent answered affirmatively, permission was requested to contact the closest in age, cancer-free, same-sex sibling living in Pennsylvania, but outside of the PWC's household. After a total of 180 siblings were interviewed no additional siblings were requested. Siblings were asked the same employment questions as the PWC and for the same time periods, namely, since the date of their matched PWCs' diagnoses, though the interviewers did not identify the date as when their sibling was diagnosed.

The use of siblings as a comparison group controlled for the social and cultural backgrounds of the respondents which could affect their problem-reporting rates. However, "contagion" may have occurred in the sense that problems reported by PWCs may have affected the siblings' problem-reporting rates. While we tried to minimize the possibility of such effects by interviewing only siblings living outside of the PWCs' households, contagion was still possible. To check on this possibility we examined whether the reporting of employment problems by PWCs and siblings were correlated and, also, whether the PWCs' medical characteristics, such as stage at diagnosis and treatments received, were related to siblings' employment problem-reporting rates.

FINDINGS

The sample differed in a number of ways from the total population of persons with cancer in the registry as a whole. There were significant differences in age (more young PWC in the sample), sex (more females in the sample), and diagnoses (more breast and fewer lung diagnoses in the sample than in the registry). These differences were due to the fact that we purposely over-sampled young persons with cancer and also to the higher death and refusal rates among certain groups of PWC. (For a more detailed discussion of the sample characteristics, see Houts et al. 1986.) To correct for these sources of bias, weighting was used to match the age, sex, and diagnostic characteristics of PWC in the registry as a whole in estimating the percent of newly diagnosed PWC having employment problems in Pennsylvania. The results are shown in Table 5.1 along with the percent of employed PWC in the sample who reported employment-related problems. Eleven

Table 5.1
Estimated Frequency of Employment Problems Among Newly
Diagnosed Persons with Cancer (PWC) Each Year in Pennsylvania

Problem	Percent of Working PWC in Sample	Estimated percent of PWC in PA
Problems Doing the Job	28%	8%
Problems in Relations With Supervisors or Co-Workers	8%	2%
Problems with Amount of Money Earned	9%	3%
Problems with Insurance Benefits from the Job	8%	2%
Problems in Keeping the Job	10%	3%
PWC Reporting at Least One Problem	39%	11%

Source: Compiled by the authors.

percent of all persons with cancer and 39 percent of PWC employed since their diagnosis reported at least one job-related problem during the period from the PWC's diagnosis. Since there are approximately 56,000 new diagnoses of cancer each year in the state, this translates to over 6000 persons with cancer each year reporting some job-related difficulties.

Next we compared employment problems reported by PWCs and their same-sex siblings. These analyses were restricted to the 90 sibling pairs where both the person with cancer and the sibling had been employed at some time since the PWCs' diagnoses. Figure 5.1 shows the results comparing the frequency with which problems were reported by both PWC and same-sex siblings since the date that the PWC was diagnosed as having cancer. Differences between the two groups were tested statistically using

Figure 5.1
Employment Problems Reported by Persons with Cancer and Their
Same-Sex Siblings

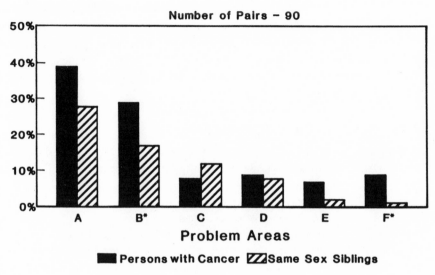

Number of Pairs – 90

Problem Areas

■ Persons with Cancer ⧅Same Sex Siblings

Source: Compiled by the authors.

the McNemar test of paired comparisons. Two statistically significant differences between the two groups were found. Significantly more PWC than
their sibling counterparts reported difficulty doing their jobs and in keeping
their jobs.

In order to assess whether problems experienced by PWC may have
affected the sibling reporting rates, the relationship between PWC characteristics and sibling reporting of employment problems were examined.
Only PWC–sibling pairs where both were working at some time since the
PWCs' diagnoses were used in these analyses. Results showed no statistical
significant associations between sibling reports of employment problems
and PWC reports of employment problems, PWC stage at diagnosis or
treatments received by PWC. Therefore, there is no indication in these data
that siblings' reporting rates were affected by their PWC siblings' problems.

Finally, logit analysis was used to determine the characteristics of PWC
most likely to report employment problems. This analysis was restricted
to persons who had worked since their diagnoses. Independent variables
were the demographic and medical characteristics of the PWC and the
dependent variable was whether a respondent had reported at least one
employment-related problem as "very much" or "some" problem. Four
characteristics were related to reporting employment problems: being
younger, having sought professional help for emotional problems prior to

the diagnosis, having received chemotherapy, and having an advanced stage of disease at diagnosis. For both age and stage at diagnosis, we examined whether there was some point at which problems were especially likely to occur. Stage of diagnosis showed approximately equal increases as stages became more serious (stage one 15%, stage two 37%, stage three 50%, and stage four 69%). Age showed a similar orderly progression with 52 percent of PWC from 20 to 39 reporting problems, 39 percent of employed PWC from 40 to 64 reporting problems, and only 21 percent of employed PWC above 64 reporting problems.

IMPLICATIONS OF THE FINDINGS

Our estimates of the frequency of reported job-related problems are somewhat smaller than those reported by Feldman (1976, 1979). She reported that 54 percent of her sample of white-collar workers and 84 percent of blue-collar workers who were employed following their diagnoses reported job-related problems because of their cancers. In part this could be because our sample was from the state registry and was adjusted to match the characteristics of all persons with cancer in the state while hers was restricted to certain age and diagnostic groups. Also, she may have included as problems events that in our study were not so scored. For example, she included, as problems, changes in assignments or working conditions that were requested by the employee and it is possible that the PWC did not see such actions as problems. Another possibility is that some events that she rated as problems were rated, by our respondents, as a "little problem" and, therefore, not scored as problems in our analyses. Finally, Feldman included problems in finding new employment while the present study did not investigate those issues.

There was considerable overlap in the extent to which PWC and their siblings reported employment-related problems. This overlap is an indication of the extent to which noncancer causes were involved in the problems experienced by PWC after their diagnoses. The overlap between PWC and their siblings is greatest for problems with supervisors and fellow workers, suggesting that interpersonal problems on the job are especially likely to involve causes in addition to the PWC's cancer. A similar finding was reported by Houts, et al. (1980), who found that PWC reports of problems with their employers following their diagnoses were significantly related to PWC reports of problems with the employer prior to their diagnoses.

The association between employment problems and chemotherapy as well as stage of disease reflects the physical effects of both the disease process and the medical treatments on PWC functioning. Earlier studies by Meyerowitz, et al. (1979, 1983) have shown that, for breast cancer patients, chemotherapy impaired general physical activity including work-related activity.

The finding that younger PWC report the more employment problems points to the special problems of younger persons in the workforce. The developmental tasks of young adulthood involve the establishment of a career direction, in addition to competence and mastery of the knowledge and skills required to advance to a chosen field. As a result, younger PWC are especially vulnerable because a serious disease, such as cancer, can have profound effects on their future in the workforce. At the same time it should also be noted that younger PWC reported higher problem rates in many areas in addition to employment (Houts et al. 1986), suggesting that younger persons may be more sensitized, in general, to the difficulties and problems associated with this illness.

CONCLUSIONS

The major finding of this study is that, while significant numbers of persons with cancer report employment problems following their diagnoses, a majority of those problems grow out of problems that are independent of the cancer. This is shown by the overlap in PWC and sibling reporting rates as well as by the associations between patient characteristics and problem reporting. The clinical significance of this is that helping PWC deal with their employment problems requires a full understanding of their work histories and work environments. Cancer care professionals should, therefore, include work histories as part of the initial psychosocial assessment as the PWC begins treatment for cancer. Work histories should include the physical requirements of a job, current job satisfaction, career goals, past and present relationships with employers, and the patient's plan as to how work responsibilities will be managed throughout treatment. This will be especially important for that population identified in this study as reporting more work problems: younger persons with cancer, with pre-existing emotional difficulties, receiving chemotherapy, and with more advanced disease.

NOTE

Support for this research was provided by the Pennsylvania Cancer Plan of the Pennsylvania Department of Health. The authors wish to thank Ivan Barofsky, Jerome Cohen, Wayne Gordon, Rochelle Habeck, William Worden, and Sandi Ezrine, for their assistance during all phases of this research. In addition, the statistical help of Charles Antle and Steven Arnold is appreciated. This chapter is adapted from the article "The incidence and causes of job-related problems among employed persons with cancer in Pennsylvania" by the same authors published in *Cancer*, 1986, *58*, 2355–2361.

REFERENCES

Feldman, F. L. *Work and cancer health histories, a study of the experiences of recovered patients.* San Francisco: American Cancer Society, California Division, 1976.

Feldman, F. L. *Work and cancer health histories, a study of the experiences of recovered blue collar workers.* San Francisco: American Cancer Society, California Division, 1978.

Greenleigh Associates, Inc. *Report on the social, economic and psychological needs of cancer patients in California.* San Francisco: American Cancer Society, California Division, 1979.

Houts, P., Lipton, A., Harvey, H., & Martin, B. Characteristics of persons who report negative work experiences following a diagnosis of cancer. Paper presented at the National Forum on Comprehensive Cancer Rehabilitation and Its Vocational Rehabilitation. Williamsburg, VA: Nov. 1980.

Houts, P., Yasko, J., Kahn, S. B., Schelzel, G., & Marconi, K. Unmet psychological, social and economic needs of persons with cancer in Pennsylvania. *Cancer,* 1986, *58,* 2355–2361.

Mellette, S. The cancer patient at work, *CA—A Cancer Journal for Clinicians,* 1985, *35,* 360–373.

Meyerowitz, B., Sparks, F., & Spears, I. Adjuvant chemotherapy for breast carcinoma: Psychosocial implications. *Cancer,* 1979, *43,* 1613–1618.

Meyerowitz, B., Watkins, R., & Sparks, F. Psychosocial implications of adjuvant chemotherapy: A two year follow up. *Cancer,* 1983, *52,* 1541–1545.

6

Work Patterns Among Long-term Survivors of Hodgkin's Disease

Patricia Fobair, Joan Bloom, Richard Hoppe, Anna Varghese, Richard Cox, and David Speigel

To every man his chance—to every man the right to live, work, to be himself, and to become whatever thing his manhood and his vision can combine to make him. (Thomas Wolfe, *You Can't Go Home Again*, 1940, p. 23)

In his view of the promise of America, Thomas Wolfe suggests to us a vision of the opportunities of life which we hold dear, opportunities which could be compromised in the case of survivors from medical casualty, such as young people recovering from Hodgkin's disease. Now that survival from cancer is improving, it is important to examine the long-term effects that cancer and its treatment may have on employment. Work and career development are essential to personal growth and the development of an individual's identity. As Feldman (1980) wrote in her study reviewing cancer health histories,

There is a deeply-entrenched tendency in our society to place a high premium on independence, both financial and psychological, and to measure the individual's adequacy with work as a means for obtaining income for meeting survival needs and improving the quality of life. . . .
Young people in our society generally grow up with the expectation that they will become earners, that on their shoulders will rest the responsibility for their own support and for that of their dependents.

What is known about the work patterns of cancer survivors? How many patients return to work following treatment? What role does the work environment play in bolstering or discouraging patients with a cancer history? What work problems or other changes occur in the employee's life following cancer treatment? In this chapter we review some recent studies including our own examination of 403 survivors of Hodgkin's disease, their work patterns and view of themselves 1–21 years after treatment at Stanford University Medical Center.

Who returns to work? Several studies in recent years have examined career patterns among young adults with cancer. Feldman (1980) studied 78 individuals treated for cancer between the ages of 13 and 23 years. She interviewed them 18 months to six years after their treatment and found that 54 percent of the patients who had been treated for lymphoma were working full-time and 18 percent part-time. In another study, Mellette (1985) found that 73 percent (22/30) of Hodgkin's disease patients had returned to work. Many find that returning to precancer employment is easier than seeking a new job. Feldman found that 69 percent of her study group returned to former employers, and 40 percent were still with their precancer work. Among those who sought new employment, 45 percent reported being rejected from at least one job, and 70 percent of these stated they were told that the diagnosis of cancer was the reason. As the number of jobs taken over the years by these patients increased, the percentage of employers told the diagnosis decreased (Feldman 1980).

The age of the patient returning to work was also an important variable. Data from Roswell Park Tumor Registry indicate that of 379 people aged 30 to 59 only 68 percent indicated that they were fully employable, while 91 percent of 132 people under the age of 29 considered themselves fully employable (Mellette 1985).

Factors related to social status and quality of the work environment have been found important in predicting work patterns. In a study of work disability among 245 patients with arthritis, Yelin et al. (1980) found that social characteristics of the workplace and the home life were more important in explaining disability outcomes than were medical variables. Economically driven factors such as the need to work, and those persons most likely to be hired explained the outcomes. Singles and other unmarried persons worked, while married persons had more choice in employment. Women and nonwhites were slightly more prone to disability, while white males were more likely to be employed. *Job prestige* was important; those with *higher status* positions, such as professionals and managers, were more likely to continue working, while service workers were more likely to stop work. As important as job prestige and social status were, qualities of the work environment, such as being able to control the pace of work, were found to be more important. Being able to take time off during the work day to receive medical care, or to decide when to take a day off without requesting a superior's permission, also increased the likelihood of staying employed (Yelin, et al. 1980).

Billings and Moos (1982) found that demographic factors and social support in the workplace were important in explaining the effects of work stress on health outcomes. They studied 360 families in a geographically defined area of San Francisco. The respondents with a positive view of their work environment were in higher level occupations, were older, more educated, and had higher incomes. They reported more employee involvement in work decision, cohesion in the work group and supervisor support, with fewer rules and less managerial control on their work. Those reporting more perceived support also reported higher levels of health and adjustment. Gender differences were found, with men benefiting from both family and work resources such as peer cohesiveness, while women were buffered more by family resources and less by work associations. While the effects of work stress on psychological functioning among men were buffered by work and family resources, they were not among women who reported higher levels of depression. Billings and Moos (1982) conclude that those persons reporting more perceived support also tend to report higher levels of health and adjustment, and that social support can attenuate the influence of work stressors on health and illness-related variables.

In a previous paper we reported that among 403 Hodgkin's disease survivors interviewed at Stanford University Medical Center, those who returned to work were more likely to be men, to report fewer symptoms of depression, and more likely to report complete return of energy (Fobair, et al. 1986).

To further explore the relationship between employment patterns, health status, and work problems, we examined these problems using a number of parameters including demographic and family roles, medical variables, work organization, and physical and emotional well-being. While we expect to find social roles and economic factors important in predicting work patterns, we believe that an even more powerful variable may be reported—physical and emotional stamina following treatment. Our hypothesis is that both return to work and fewer problems reported at work will related to the individuals' having a complete return of energy following treatment as well as having a positive view of themselves.

METHODS

These data come from a cross-sectional survey of patients who were treated on several prospective randomized clinical trails for Hodgkin's disease at Stanford University Medical Center (Fobair, et al. 1986). All patients returning for regular follow-up were invited to participate in the study. Four hundred and three agreed (a 95% response rate). A self-administered

Table 6.1
Characteristics of Hodgkin's Disease Study Population

CHARACTERISTICS	NUMBER	PERCENT
Gender: Male	222	55
Female	181	45
Stage I-II	242	60
III-IV	161	40
Treatment		
XRT Alone	151	38
XRT + Chemo	207	51
XRT + Chemo for Relapse	27	7
Chemo Only	18	5
Current Status		
No Relapse	333	83
Relapse Currently No Disease	63	16
Relapse with Disease	7	2

XRT - Irradiation

Chemo - Chemotherapy

Source: Compiled by the authors.

questionnaire was given during the regularly scheduled follow-up visits followed by an interview by a clinical social worker or a medical student.

The characteristics for the study population are summarized in Table 6.1. The age of the subjects at the time of treatment was 27.4 years (range 5–65). The age at the time of interview was 36.3 years (range 15–78). The median duration of follow-up was nine years (range 1–21 years). Sixty percent of the patients had been treated for limited (stage I–II) disease. The initial treatments used included combined modality therapy with radiation and chemotherapy (52% of patients), radiation therapy alone (45%) (7% of patients later received chemotherapy for relapse) and chemotherapy alone (7%). At the time of interview, 82 percent of the patients had never relapsed, 16 percent had relapsed but were without evidence of disease after salvage therapy, and 2 percent of the patients had active disease. The type of treatment correlated highly with stage of disease.

The data for these analyses were derived from questions designed to assess disruption in employment, family relationships, and sense of well-being. Standard survey items were used to describe occupational prestige, marital status, and perception of health. Items developed by Barofsky (1978) were used to assess work relationships and job discrimination. Questions concerned number of hours worked per week, description of occupation, usual job title and number of years in that work, difficulties at work due to medical history, inability to take jobs due to health condition, lack of opportunities in work selection due to Hodgkin's disease, personal view of ambition for career, and employer's knowledge of medical history. Questions were designed specifically for this study to evaluate potential disruptions in family and intimate relationships. Social status was assessed using Hollingshead's Four Factor Index. Specially designed questions were utilized to assess alteration of energy level and changes in physical activity. Patients were asked if their energy level had changed and, if it had, how long it took to return to normal. While these data are subject to bias due to memory, reliability checks were carried out on 35 percent of the sample. Self-esteem was measured using Rosenberg's scale (Rosenberg 1965). The CES-D, a 20-item standardized scale, was used to assess depression. This scale was selected as items do not mimic the experience of physical illness. It provides a measure that has been developed for use with a normal population. Reliability and validity studies for the CES-D have been conducted and normative data for both institutionalized and community populations are available for comparison (Radloff 1977; Sayetta & Johnson 1980).

Relationships among variables were analyzed by means of standard statistical methods (Mendenhall 1979), including contingency tables, students t-test, and linear regression.

RESULTS

Patterns of Employment

Who worked and who did not? As reported previously (Fobair, et al. 1986), 54 percent were working 40 or more hours per week, 17 percent were working less than 40 hours, and 29 percent were unemployed. Men were significantly more likely to be working than women, regardless of age or marital pattern, while younger women, more often unmarried and without children, were more likely than older women to be working (see Table 6.2).

What career patterns did they occupy in the employment world? Among the 367 (91%) who provided us with a job description, 62 or 17 percent were employed as executives; owners of large or medium size businesses;

Table 6.2

Employment Status of Male and Female Respondents

EMPLOYMENT	TOTAL N	%	MALE N	%	FEMALE N	%
Full Employment (40 or more hours/week)	216	(54)	164	(74)	52	(29)
Part Time Employment (0-40 hours/week)	70	(17)	18	(8)	52	(29)
Unemployed	116	(29)	40	(18)	76	(42)
TOTAL	403	(100)	222	(55)	181	(45)

* Patients > 16 years

Source: Compiled by authors.

professionals such as attorneys, physicians, architects, or administrators; or teachers. A middle group of 232 patients (63%) (score of 4–7 on Hollingshead social status schedule) occupied positions in the middle range of job prestige, such as farm owners, managers, technicians, owners of small businesses, clerical and sales workers or skilled craftsmen. At the lower end of the scale (scores 1–3 Hollingshead) were 73 patients (20%) who held semi-skilled or unskilled positions such as farm workers, bus drivers, file clerks, newsboys, and dishwashers (see Table 6.3).

Issues involved in quality of work, the type of job, and the physical demands of the job, were related to being employed. Of 367 patients who reported their occupation, we compared each gender for work relating to things, people, and need for strength. Women were more likely to have jobs where they worked with office equipment ($t = 2.7$; $df = 365$; $P = 0.006$), while men were more likely to have work that required physical strength ($t = 8.5$; $df = 365$; $P = 0.0001$). There was a more statistically significant ($t = 1.7$; $df = 365$; $P = 0.08$) trend for men to be more involved with people in their work. (The 36 patients who did not provide job information were usually homemakers with minimal work experience, or students who may have worked sporadically.)

Following treatment, people holding jobs with higher occupational prestige worked longer hours ($t = 3.6$; $df = 341$; $P = 0.0004$). These findings held even after controlling for the effects of age and time since treatment. When men and women were examined separately, younger women and those further from treatment worked longer hours.

Table 6.3
Occupational Status of Hodgkin's Disease Respondents

OCCUPATIONAL STATUS	N	%
(9)* Professionals (including executive officers)	32	8
(8) Administrators	30	7
(7) Managers	45	11
(6) Technicians/Semi Professional	71	18
(5) Clerical & Sales	38	9
(4) Small Business	78	20
(3) Semi Skilled Worker	46	11
(2) Unskilled Labor	20	5
(1) Farm Labor	7	2
(0) No Job Code	36	9
TOTAL	403	100

*Higher number implies higher status (Hollingshead, 1950).
Source: Compiled by authors, according to A. B. Hollingshead, four factor index of social status, working paper, 1950.

Unemployment

At the time of the interview, 286 patients were working; 117 patients were unemployed. Of the 117 patients who were not employed, women outnumbered men (76 women, 41 men), the largest subgroup of the unemployed were (29) married women "managing households." Another subgroup of 21 people "looking for work," were married and there were an equal number of men and women. Of the 14 patients on "permanent disability," most were married men (78%). Five women described themselves as "volunteers" and most of them were married, as were those patients who marked their employment status as "other" (seven people had never worked).

About 40 percent of the unemployed (46 patients), were students, those who indicated they were looking for work, or others who had recently finished treatment and might be expected to return to work in the near future. The group *not* expected to return to work included 70 persons who managed households, had retired, or were disabled. Most of this group had not worked for two or more years. It could be assumed that these 70 patients (17% of the 403 patients) probably would not return to the world of employment. In summary, with the exception of students, most of the unemployed were married.

The characteristics of those 258 (64%) individuals who worked 20 hours per week or more differed in some ways from those 146 (36%) who were working less than 20 hours or were unemployed. In assessing this dichotomy, the following psychological parameters were predictive.

Predictors of Employment

Medical

State of disease, treatment, and medical status at the time of interview were examined in relation to working hours at the time of interview. As previously indicated (Fobair, et al. 1986), 60 percent presented with early stage (I–II) disease, and 40 percent with later stages (III–IV). Treatment included adjuvant chemotherapy with radiation (51%), radiation therapy alone (38%), radiation with chemotherapy for relapse disease (7%), and chemotherapy alone (5%). At the time of interview, 82 percent of the patients were without evidence of disease, and among the 18 percent who experienced relapse, only 2 percent remained with disease after treatment. One might expect that patients with later stage disease, more extensive treatment, or relapsing disease to be among those who worked less, yet we did not find this so. Work patterns were not directly affected by medical or treatment variables.

Demography

How did the effects of having had Hodgkin's disease impact the work patterns by gender or age group? Gender was very powerful in predicting who was working at the time of interview. Women were less frequently working full-time. Younger women (less than 30 years) were more likely to work. Women over the age of 30 at the time of interview were more likely to have one or more children ($x^2 = 9.16$; df $= 1$; P $< .002$).

Social Roles

Being married, having children, having more education, and holding jobs with greater occupational prestige were related to employment patterns at the time of the interview. Over two-thirds of the patients were married or living as married at the time of the interview, equally distributed between men and women. Marital status was more likely to predict women's employment (P $= 0.08$), than men's employment. Consistent with established social roles, married women were less likely to work than unmarried women ($x^2 = 69.04$; df $= 1$; P $< .000001$). Having one or more children was the most predictive factor differentiating women who worked and those who didn't ($x^2 < 3.6$; df $= 1$; P < 0.06), while more college-educated women

(43%) stayed home after treatment than college-educated men (12%); this can be explained by the women's marital status and number of dependents.

We examined social status and work patterns and defining social status according to the Hollingshead's Four Factor Index (education, gender, marital status, and occupational patterns), we found that seventy-eight patients (19%) were in the highest social strata, major business and professional people. One-hundred fifty-six patients (39%) described their careers as medium size business, minor professional, and technical work. In the remaining three strata were 103 (26%) skilled craftsmen, 59 semi-skilled workers (15%), and five unskilled persons (1%). When social status scores were evaluated for each gender, women's scores were not significantly higher than men's (women's score 42.8, men's score 41.7). Men who were employed at the time of the interview were more likely to be of higher social status than unemployed men (t = 1.96; df = 201; P < .05).

Working Roles

Work patterns were assessed by a number of parameters including job prestige, co-worker support, adequacy of finances, and quality of the work environment.

For this analysis, housewives whose unemployment might be expected were eliminated from the sample. These included women over 66 and under 20 years of age at the time of the interview. The remaining men and women (n = 341) were compared by the number of hours worked per week (workers full-time), plus those who worked more than 20 hours per week with those who worked less than 20 hours per week. Patients with greater job prestige tended to work more than 20 hours per week (t = 3.59; df = 341; P = 0.0004). Co-worker support was also higher for patients working 20 hours per week or more than for those working less than 20 hours (t = 11.4; df = 341; P = 0.0000). Co-worker support was more important for women than men. Full-time working women, reported more support than part-time workers (t = 1.85; df = 103; P = 0.07). Among the men there were no differences (P = 0.94).

Patients over 30 reported more co-worker support than those less than 30 years of age (t = 2.5; df = 341; P = 0.0004). Co-worker support was greater for those with more job prestige (t = 3.91; df = 341; P = 0.002). While social status did not predict work hours, co-worker support and social status were correlated (t = 2.51; df = 341; P = 0.01).

How did study participants view the adequacy of their finances? Men working less than 20 hours per week were less at ease about adequacy of finances than those employed full-time (t = 2.17; df = 212; P = 0.03). Men working less than 20 hours per week were also more distressed about inadequate finances than women working less than 20 hours per week (t = 1.9; df = 118; P = 0.04). Even if retired or disabled from illness, unemployed men worried more about finances than did women.

Feeling Fit

Energy, activities, and ambition to work were important areas of examination in understanding work patterns. As reported previously, patients whose energy had not returned were less likely to be working (t = 3.96; df = 401; P = 0.00025). Men who were employed less than 20 hours per week were significantly more likely to report that their energy did not return following treatment (x^2 = 7.08; df = 1; P = 0.008). While energy return was important for women who returned to work 20 hours or more per week at the time of the interview, it was less important than for the men (x^2 = 4.8; df = 1; P = 0.03).

Among the 271 patients who reported working more than 20 hours per week, 185 or 68 percent felt well, and reported energy return, but 86 (32%) people reported less optimal energy return, and they also were working 20 hours or more. Examined by gender, more of the men, 71 percent of those whose energy had not returned to normal were working while 39 percent of the women whose energy had not returned to normal were working. Only 13 percent of the men whose energy had returned were not working, while 43 percent of the women whose energy had returned were not working. The society view of womens' roles, especially for those who are married with children, gave more flexibility in choosing to work or not. For both genders, energy return was important in explaining employment (t = −4.86; df = 2,64; P = 0.0000). A lack of return of energy correlated with those patients who did not work (t = 5.4; df = 125; P < 0.0001). Social status among the 271 employed patients differed by reports of return of energy. There was a difference in social status between the 185 whose energy had returned versus those who worked with less energy return (t = 1.96; df = 269; P = 0.05). There were no differences in social status by energy return among the patients who were not working.

Ambition is not a requirement of working, it is more subtle, a quality or attitude which when felt encourages drive, or incentive for advancement. An indicator of energy, ambition and energy are words involved in the definition of the other. Yet, ambition is the result of choice, while energy is closer to a feeling of power or activity level. Patients were asked if they felt more or less ambitious about their work as a result of their diagnosis or treatment for Hodgkin's disease: 53 percent (213) felt about the same, 25 percent (102) felt more, and 18 percent (72) felt less ambition. Comparing ambition with other predictor variables we found the patient's view to be important in describing other major outcomes.

While patient scores of ambition were not directly related to type of treatment, ambition scores went down as stage of disease went up (x^2 = 68; df = 1; P = 0.01). Patients who had treatment for recurrent disease reported a reduction in their ambition (P = 0.04), compared to patients without evidence of disease.

Being younger than 30 at the time of diagnosis and at the interview were related to increased ambition. Those who were less than 30 at diagnosis reported greater ambition ($x^2 = 9.4$; df $= 1$; P $= 0.01$), as did those who were under 30 at the time of the interview ($x^2 = 8.2$; df $= 1$; P $= 0.004$). Recently treated patients did not feel as ambitious as those further away in years from treatment (t $= 3.6$; df $= 251$; P $= 0.0004$), and less ambitious patients did not work as many hours per week as patients who felt more ambitious ($x^2 = 4.7$; df $= 1$; P $= 0.03$). Just as the number of hours worked was lower for those feeling less ambition ($x^2 = 9.3$; df $= 1$; P $= 0.002$).

Patient reports of being able to resume normal activities were correlated with working more ($x^2 = 5.7$; df $= 1$; P $= 0.02$), especially for men ($x^2 = 3.5$; df $= 1$; P $= 0.06$). In terms of feeling fit, energy, changes in ambition, and the ability to maintain normal activities were each important to predicting employment.

A Personal View of Oneself

Body image, self-esteem, depression, and problems requiring counseling were a group of variables that interconnected with each other and predicted hours worked. Body image is central to a picture we have of our physical well-being. Patients who worked more hours per week were more likely to report a positive view of their body image than those who didn't ($x^2 = 6.4$; df $= 1$; P $= 0.01$). Working men were more likely to report a better body image than nonworking men ($x^2 = 4.6$; df $= 1$; P $= 0.03$), though working did not predict women's scores. Feeling that one's body image was back to normal was related to having better energy return ($x^2 = 17.7$; df $= 1$; P $= 0.00003$), fewer symptoms of depression (t $= 5.22$; df $= 301$; P $= 0.000011$), and greater ambition ($x^2 = 7.5$; df $= 1$; P $= 0.006$). Yet, body image and two other variables interacted in a curious way, perhaps indicating the vulnerability to change that this factor encompasses. Higher status, better educated patients were more likely to report greater negative changes in body image than those from lower status positions (t $= -2.4$; df $= 399$; P $= 0.02$); and people with later stage disease were more likely to report lower body image ($x^2 = 6.5$; df $= 1$; P $= 0.01$).

At the time of the interview, patients were asked to evaluate their self-esteem. Their individual self-esteem scores were highly correlated to the number of hours they worked (t $= 3.3$; df $= 386$; P $= 0.001$), the amount of co-worker support they had (t $= 2.9$; df $= 386$; P $= 0.004$), the return of feelings of energy (t $= 3.2$; df $= 404$; P $= 0.002$), and being less depressed (t $= 3.5$; df $= 382$; P $= 0.0005$). Thus, self-esteem was highly correlated with patients' evaluations of themselves, their work, and their energy.

Absence of symptoms of depression (t $= 3.96$; df $= 401$; P $= 0.0002$) and problems that required counseling ($x^2 = 6.2$; df $= 1$; P $= 0.01$) were

Table 6.4
Effect of Social and Demographic Factors on Hours Worked Using Multiple Regression

SOCIAL FACTORS	REGRESSION COEFFICIENT	T-TEST	P-VALUE
Co-worker Support			
Low vs. High	1.21	8.92	10^6
Gender: Female vs. Male	10.46	5.87	10^6
Depression			
CES-D $\geq$ 16 v. CES-D < 16	-0.37	-3.66	.00032
Body Image			
Less Attractive vs. Same	5.59	2.77	.006

$r^2 =.37$ F=45.1   P <.001

Source: Compiled by the authors, based on multiregression technique of Cox (1972).

also related to hours worked. Hours spent at work was not related to gender or age; however, each variable was highly correlated with energy and ambition. Both might be considered results of the person's life experience to this point of time. Both depression (t = 3.7; df = 393; P = 0.0002) and ambition for work (x^2 = 4.8; df = 1; P = 0.02) got better as time post-treatment increased. This may be the result of less worry and greater energy.

As 15 variables were correlated with the number of hours worked, multivariate linear regression was used to determine the best fit model for number of hours worked (see Table 6.4). The most predictive model contained co-worker support, gender, depression, and body image. The total model explained 37 percent of the variance. For men, three variables were significant predictors (Table 6.5): more co-worker support, less depression and better body image. For women, the regression revealed a slightly different pattern (Table 6.5): more co-worker support, younger age at treatment, and less depression. The best fit model for men explained less variance than the one for women (25 percent compared to 40 percent).

Work Problems

Questions asked about work problems included concerns about job discrimination, problems with job seeking, withdrawing from work, or failure to accept promotion due to illness or treatment experiences. There were

Table 6.5

Effect of Social and Demographic Factors on Hours Worked, by Gender

SOCIAL FACTOR	MALES		
	COEFFICIENT	T-TEST	P VALUES
Co-worker Support	0.95	5.3	0.000001
Depression	-0.44	-3.3	.002
Body Image	-6.27	-2.3	.03
	r^2-.25	F-20.5	P-<.01

r^2 .25 for men

SOCIAL FACTOR	FEMALES		
	COEFFICIENT	T-TEST	P VALUES
Co-worker Support	1.48	7.2	0.000001
Depression	0.44	2.8	.006
Younger Age	-0.29	2.1	.04
	r^2-.40	F-26.6	P-<.01

r^2 .40 for women

Source: Compiled by the authors.

493 instances of work difficulty reported by 258 patients (64%). Over one-third of the patients reported "no problems" (145 patients, 36%). Using Heilman's "Lack-of-Fit Model" (Barofsky, Chapter 1, this volume), we found that 173 of the patients or 67 percent of those with problems believed that they had been negatively evaluated by others in job selection, lost benefits following their illness and recurring adverse performance appraisal for advancement, while 85 patients (33%) limited their own job options for career advancement due to their disease or treatment of Hodgkin's disease (see Figure 6.1).

Self-limited career options was the most frequently mentioned problem (157 instances, 32%), followed by loss of benefits (149 instances, 30%), adverse job selection (99 instances, 20%), adverse appraisal (46 instances, 10%), and self-limited career advancement (42 instances, 8%).

The characteristics of the 258 patients who reported work problems were

Figure 6.1
Distribution of Hodgkin's Disease Patients by Number of Problems:
Lack-of-Fit Model and Job Discrimination

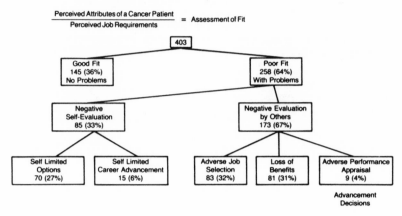

Adaptation of Figure 1, Heilman, *Research in Organizational Behavior*, 1983, *5*, p. 281.

compared to the 145 who reported "no" problems. Higher stage disease, loss of energy, few activities, less ambition, poor coping skills, a negative body image, lower self-esteem, higher scores of depression, and receiving counseling for emotional problems were positively correlated with experiencing work problems.

Patients who were diagnosed with higher stage Hodgkin's disease at the time of treatment were more likely to report work problems at the time of interview ($x^2 = 8.4$; df = 1; P = 0.0004). Patients who stated that their energy had not returned to normal, were more likely to report work problems ($x^2 = 15.2$; df = 1; P = 0.0001). Feeling less fit frequently meant fewer normal activities were continued during treatment and thereafter. Those who reported being less able to maintain moderate activity levels were also most likely to report work problems ($x^2 = 3.99$; df = 1; P = 0.05). Patients who enumerated one or more work problems were more likely to report "lower ambition" at the time of the interview compared with those who did not report work problems ($x^2 = 9.1$; df = 1; P = 0.003).

Examining the factors that describe one's personal view of oneself, patients whose coping skills were more passive were also more likely to report work problems (t = 3.3; df = 341; P = 0.001). Intercorrelated with coping skills were patient self-ratings of self-esteem, body image, energy level, depression scores, and counseling for emotional problems. Patients who reported less of a positive view of their body image were also more likely to experience work problems ($x^2 = 4.5$; df = 1; P = 0.0001). While patient scores of self-esteem were generally high, those who reported less positive

Table 6.6
Effect of Body Image, Perceived Energy Return, and Emotional
Problems on the Number of Reported Work Problems

SOCIAL FACTOR	REGRESSION COEFFECIENT	T TEST	P VALUE
Body Image	0.16	2.79	0.006
Worst View vs. Better View			
Energy Return	0.14	2.72	0.007
Less vs. More			
Counseling for Emotional Problems	0.17	2.55	0.01
More vs. Less			

$$r^2 = .09 \quad F=11.02 \quad P=0.01$$

Source: Compiled by the authors.

self-esteem also reported work problems (t = 2.38; df = 396; P = 0.02). Patients with higher scores of depression reported work problems more often than those with lower scores (t = 2.7; df = 386; P = 0.007). And those patients who received counseling for emotional problems were also more likely to report work problems (x^2 = 11.13; df = 1; P = 0.001).

Multiple regression analysis revealed that counseling for emotional problems, negative changes in body image, and loss of energy significantly accounted for the number of work problems (see Table 6.6). This analysis accounted for 9 percent of the variance for men (body image and counseling for emotional problems were most predictive), while for women loss of energy was the key predictor to work problems (see Table 6.7).

Employers and others might explain problems on the job to be a function of the individual's social problems which are unrelated to their cancer. Such problems might include drinking and drug use. Thus, in order to see if job discrimination does exist, we wanted to rule out these alternative explanations. Only 29 people (7%) reported a history of problems with alcohol or drugs; work problems were unrelated to such a history. Those patients with work problems did not differ from those without problems in relation to alcohol intake.

"Telling the employer" about having had Hodgkin's disease was investigated. Two-thirds of the 182 patients whose diagnosis occurred prior to their current employment decided to tell their employer about their diag-

Table 6.7
Effects of Body Image, Perceived Energy Return and Emotional Problems on Work Problems Reported by Males and Females

SOCIAL FACTOR	MALES			FEMALES		
	COEFFICIENT	T-TEST	P VALUE	COEFFICIENT	T-TEST	P VALUE
Body Image						
Worse view vs. Better View	0.19	2.4	0.02	0.14	1.6	ns
Energy Return						
Less vs. More	0.70	1.0	ns	0.24	2.9	.005
Counseling Emotional Problems						
More vs. Less	0.19	2.08	0.04	0.15	1.6	ns
	r^2=.11	F=5.4	P=.01	r^2=.13	F=2.7	P=.01

Source: Compiled by the authors.

nosis. In 170 instances (42%), the diagnosis was made after current employment began. Only 60 patients (15%) concealed their cancer history from their employers.

DISCUSSION

In this analysis of the work patterns of 403 Hodgkin's disease patients, the individual's support system at work, their mood and personal view of self were more important in explaining work patterns than physical limitations caused by the disease and/or its treatment.

Like the patterns studied by Feldman (1980) and Mellette (1985), a majority (71%) of our patients were working full- or part-time at the time of the interview. The unemployed in our study were likely to be housewives caring for children in the home, or students looking for work, or less often those who were disabled and retired.

Like Mellette (1985), we found age (less than 30 years at the time of diagnosis, and at the interview) to be important in predicting employment but only for women. The men in our group worked regardless of age.

Single women were most likely to be employed, married women with children least likely. Individuals with higher job prestige, better education, and greater social status were more likely to be employed than those at lower ends of the scale. Of all the factors considered, co-worker support was the most powerful predictor of the number of work hours (see Table 6.4). Like Yelin, et al. (1980) we did not find that medical variables explained work patterns. As described in Table 6.4, positive co-worker support, male gender, less depression, and a positive view of one's body image were important predictors of the number of hours our patients worked.

These findings are consistent with the results of our analysis (Fobair, et al. 1986), where gender and depression were important covariates. Now co-worker support and body image join the group of independent variables found to be predictors. Younger age for women, having greater energy return, and remaining active continue to show correlation with work hours but are not as predictive as co-worker support, gender, mood, and one's view of body image.

In an expanded analysis of work problems we found 493 instances of self-reported work problems among 64 percent of the Hodgkin's disease patients. This is higher than our previous report of 42 percent among 168 patients (Fobair, et al. 1986). The results (64%) now fall closer to the number of patients with work problems discussed in Feldman's work, where 54 percent of the white-collar patients experienced one or more work problems, while 84 percent of the blue-collar patients reported such problems (Feldman 1980).

Evaluating the kind of work problems experienced by patients, we utilized Barofsky's adaptation of Heilman's Lack-of-Fit Model of Discrimination (Chapter 1, this volume). Sixty-seven percent of the 258 patients with problems described them as a result of "negative evaluation by others," such as adverse job selection, and loss of benefits. Yet, the single problem cited most frequently was "self-limited career option," noted by 157 patients (32%).

Examining the variables associated with work problems is also illuminating. Although one-to-one correlations with medical variables showed significance for those who reported work problems, the multiple regression suggested three important psychosocial variables; a history of counseling for emotional problems; feeling a negative perception of one's body image; and lack of energy return. Men who reported work problems were more likely to report that counseling had been needed, and to perceive negative changes in body image, while women with work problems were more likely to report losses in energy.

These findings suggest areas of educational and emotional support in the treatment setting. Although work patterns after cancer appear more determined by prior demographic and social status characteristics, the additionally significant psychosocial variables—activity, depression, and body image—suggest areas for counseling or educational support. Encouraging activities as energy permits during treatment may be more therapeutic for patients than "understanding" their loss of energy and sympathizing with their increased need for sleep; maintaining physical activity may prevent negative changes later on in body image. Assisting patients in finding suitable one-to-one or group therapy for treatment of depression may also be an area for greater emphasis in our contacts with cancer patients.

We have recently begun a modest pilot program with the physical therapy programs at Stanford University Hospital. Patients are encouraged to consider more active physical activity. When patients are interested, we refer them to physical therapy for an evaluation and treatment plan. Their current strength and activity level is tested and a program outlined which will increase their overall muscle tone and strength. Many patients have used the program and have later reported that their energy and activity levels did not diminish during or after treatment. Thus, the loss of energy reported of many patients may be due to decreased activity during the treatment of Hodgkin's disease rather than a side effect of the treatment.

Vulnerability to work problems seems somewhat higher for those with later stage disease and greater need for more extensive treatment. As physicians, social workers, and others, we can be alert to these possibilities, and willing to talk about them with patients. Whenever possible, counseling and patient support problems that reinforce problem solving could strengthen the coping techniques of patients and families. The task for many patients is finding a way not to feel like a victim. This involves mastery of illness-related issues and attending to former tasks of life as well.

The adaptive issue after treatment is complicated and includes maintaining continuity: "finding a way to return to the fabric of one's life after the dislocation of illness and treatment" (Mages, et al. 1981). The adaptive task is to understand and communicate one's changed attitudes, needs, and limitations so that a new balance can be formed with the environment (Barofsky 1981). Our experience in the clinical setting is that when former patients are still worried about other issues, such as the possibility of recurrence and progression of disease, or damage to one's body from the illness or treatment, or when they haven't had sufficient opportunity to work through the trauma of the acute illness as it occurred, initially they sometimes become constricted in their activities, or assume an identity based on being a "cancer patient" (Fobair, et al. 1981).

Self-help, education, or support groups can be helpful to both patients undergoing therapy and those returning for follow-up who are interested in talking about these issues. At Stanford, we have found that a small group (6–8) of patients with Hodgkin's disease want to meet and talk about their experiences while they are undergoing therapy. A regular group of 8–12 follow-up patients meets monthly to discuss the issues that they are facing in their lives after treatment is completed.

Referrals to state vocational rehabilitation programs have been helpful to many patients. We have developed a good, working relationship with the office nearest our institution. This has permitted patients to become acquainted with their services and programs before they were physically ready for referral to the offices in their hometown. Some women who were housewives before treatment have decided to finish their education or seek full-time employment after treatment ends. Some younger men decided to change career direction as a result of value changes experienced during treatment. Disruptions in the normal flow of employment occur in many forms. Patients with less education and fewer resources may be more vulnerable to work problems than others. In the San Francisco Bay area, we have a special section of the Legal Aid Society who help the disabled with employment discrimination problems. Funded in part from the American Cancer Society, this group writes a newsletter, "ACCESS," which is designed to assist people at many different levels to learn their rights in the employment world.

SUMMARY

In conclusion, our hypotheses were partially supported. We expected to find that while social roles and economic factors were important in predicting work patterns, emotional and physical stamina would be even more powerful in predicting return to work and work problems. We found that social support at work, male gender, less depression, and a better body image were predictors of work patterns. Work problems after cancer were predicted by variables descriptive of physical and emotional stamina, and were not influenced by biological, demographic or social and work roles. Social service programs for patients in treatment and returning for follow-up medical visits are encouraged. Individual and group meetings can be helpful. Referrals to state agency rehabilitation programs and legal aid programs can also be supportive.

To paraphrase Thomas Wolfe, we were happy to find that, for most of our patients, there was the chance to live, to work, to be themselves, and usually to become whatever their visions could combine to make them, while for those with difficulty, there was help to assist them in finding remedies in the environment and within themselves.

REFERENCES

Barofsky, I. Unpublished research, 1978.

Barofsky, I. Job description of cancer patients: What we know and what we need to know. Paper presented at the American Cancer Society, Virginia Division, March 1981.

Barofsky, I. Work: Issues and concepts. In I. Barofsky (Ed.), *Work and illness: The cancer patient.* New York: Praeger, 1989, pp. 3–24.

Billings, A. G., & Moos, R. H. Work stress and the stress buffering roles of work and family resources. *Occupational Behavior,* 1982, *3,* 215–232.

Cox, D. R. Regression models and life tables. *Journal of the Royal Statistical Society* (B), 1972, *34,* 187–220.

Feldman, F. *Work and cancer health histories: Work expectations and experiences in youth (ages 13–23) with cancer histories.* San Francisco: American Cancer Society, California Division, 1980.

Fobair, P., Wolfson, A., Mages, N., Hall, J., Harrison, J., & Jose, J. Psychosocial aspects of radiation therapy. In P. Tretter, L. Leinger, A. Keitscher, R. Torpie, R. DeBellis, & M. Fallmer (Eds.), *Group work with cancer patients in radiation therapy.* New York: Arno Press, 1981.

Fobair, P., Hoppe, R. T., Bloom, J., Cox, R., Varghese, A., & Speigel, D. Psychosocial problems among survivors of Hodgkin's disease. *Journal of Clinical Oncology,* 1986, *4,* 805–814.

Hollingshead, A. B. Four factor index of social status. Working paper, 1950.

Mages, N., Mendlesohn, G., & Castro, J. Concepts of adaptation and life change in cancer patients. Psychosocial aspects of radiation therapy. In P. Tretter, L. Liegner, A. Keitscher, R. Torpie, R. DeBellis, & M. Fallmer (Eds.), *Group work with cancer patients in radiation therapy.* New York: Arno Press, 1981.

Mellette, S. The cancer patient at work. *CA—A Cancer Journal for Clinicians,* 1985, *36,* 360–373.

Mendenhall, W. *Introduction to probability and statistics.* 5th ed. North Scituate, MA: PWS Publishers, 1979, pp. 277–401.

Radloff, L. CES-D scale: A self-report depression scale for research in the general population. *Applied Psychological Measurement,* 1977, *1,* 385–401.

Rosenberg, M. *Society and the adolescent self-image.* Princeton, NJ: Princeton University Press, 1965.

Sayetta, R. B., & Johnson, D. P. Basic data on depressive symptomatology. Vital and Health Statistical Series 11, Number 216, 1980. National Center for Health Statistics. USHEW CDHEW-PHS80–1666, pp. 1–31.

Yelin, E., Nevitt, M., & Epstein, W. Toward an epidemiology of work disability. *Milbank Memorial Fund Quarterly. Health and Society*, 1980, *58*, 386–415.

7

Information about Work from Studies with the Cancer Inventory of Problem Situations (CIPS)

Patricia A. Ganz, Cyndie Coscarelli Schag, and Richard L. Heinrich

Advances in the treatment of cancer have led to higher cure rates and lengthened survival times for individuals who develop one of the many neoplastic disorders called cancer. Similar to heart disease, cancer has become a chronic illness for many patients, frequently manifested by a series of exacerbations and remissions. However, the therapies used in the treatment of cancer are frequently more intensive and toxic than for other serious or chronic illnesses. Psychological and social concerns may play an important role in the cancer patient's adaptation to this chronic illness. Societal and individual fears about cancer as a disease may influence the subsequent rehabilitation of some cancer patients.

Surprisingly, few studies have examined the relationship between cancer and the ability to work (Feldman 1976, 1978, 1980; Greenleigh Associates 1979). Recent improvements in cancer patient survival during the last decade make this area of research more meaningful (Mellette 1985). The studies of Feldman have pioneered in this arena (Feldman 1976, 1978, 1980). The interview data from her studies are rich in descriptive material, which captures the positive and negative aspects of the work experience as perceived by cancer patients, their physicians, and their employers. Indirectly these studies examine discrimination in employment practices related to cancer patients. From these studies one concludes that blue-collar workers experience more work-related problems than the white-collar respondents, and that, in general, young cancer patients experience the fewest problems (Feldman 1976, 1978, 1980).

Additional information about work and cancer comes from research sponsored by the American Cancer Society, California Division, Inc. (Greenleigh Associates 1979). This study examined a sample of 810 cancer patients, predominantly white and female in late middle age or older, who were diagnosed during the period July 1, 1975, to June 30, 1976. Interviews with these patients were conducted between six and 24 months after the cancer diagnosis, with emphasis on demographic and socioeconomic characteristics of the patient, problems and changes that occurred in relation to the diagnosis, treatment and recovery from the cancer, and the availability of social services to assist in meeting the perceived problems or needs. This survey revealed a decline in full-time employment for the respondents which was related to the specific cancer site. There was an increase in part-time employment, disability, and retirement for all cancer sites. When these principal activities were examined according to age, the greatest change occurred in the subjects aged 46–64 years. In addition, there was a positive correlation between income level at the time of cancer diagnosis and continued employment at the time of interview (Greenleigh Associates 1979).

Our research has focused on the psychosocial and rehabilitation needs of cancer patients living with cancer as a chronic disease (Heinrich, Schag, & Ganz 1984; Schag, Heinrich, & Ganz 1983). We have collected information from a cross-section of patients using a cancer-specific self-report survey questionnaire, the Cancer Inventory of Problem Situations (CIPS), along with detailed medical, social, and demographic information (Schag, et al. 1983). The Karnofsky Performance Status (KPS) scale (Karnofsky & Burchenal 1949; Schag, Heinrich, & Ganz 1984), the most common measure of functional performance used in oncologic practice, has been utilized in the evaluation of all of our subjects. In developing his performance status scale, Karnofsky closely linked the ability to work and carry out daily activities as a functional correlate of disease activity (Karnofsky, et al. 1949). Subsequently, many clinical studies have shown a close association between the KPS and the length of an individual patient's survival (Stanley 1980; Berry 1979). Ratings of this scale directly relate to the ability to work (and indirectly to the extent of disease). Therefore, the KPS may be helpful to measure for adjustment of a wide variety of physical and medical problems related to the cancer and its treatment which may impact on the cancer patient's ability to work. This chapter reviews our studies with the CIPS in relation to work, with particular emphasis on the medical and demographic factors that may affect the ability to work.

METHOD

Instruments

The Cancer Inventory of Problem Situations (CIPS)

The CIPS is a recently developed cancer-specific survey instrument which contains 144 statements which describe the problems faced by cancer patients as they live day-to-day with the disease (Heinrich, et al. 1984; Schag, et al. 1983). Patients are instructed to read each statement and decide on the degree to which it applies to their situation within the past month. The response is rated on a five-point scale ranging from "not at all" to "very much." The problems are divided into broad categories which include functional health status, difficulty communicating with the medical team, chemotherapy-related problems, communication at work, worry, cognitive problems, problems obtaining information from the medical team, discomfort during medical procedures, job-related problems, difficulty interacting with friends and relatives, anxiety in medical situations, communication with partner, affection, sexual dysfunction, interaction with partner, and dating for those who are single. The reliability, validity, and acceptability of this instrument have been studied in a heterogeneous sample of 306 cancer patients (Schag, et al. 1983).

Background Information Form

This form is completed by each subject at the same time the CIPS is administered. Information requested includes age, sex, education, occupation, current household income, marital status, work status (yes or no), time since last worked, religious preference, ethnicity, number of household members, and number of children.

Medical Summary Sheet

This form is completed by the patient's physician or a research assistant at the time the CIPS is administered. Specific medical information is requested that describes the extent of the patient's disease at the time of diagnosis, the patient's current care status (no evidence of disease, locally recurrent, or extensive disease), how long the patient has been in this care status, whether the patient currently has metastatic disease, the type of prior treatment and the current treatment (surgery, chemotherapy, or radiation), and the goals of therapy (curative, long-term control, or palliative).

Karnofsky Performance Status (KPS)

Since its introduction in 1949, the KPS has been used increasingly to evaluate therapeutic outcome, to stratify patients in clinical trials, and as a guide to treatment planning (Karnofsky, et al. 1949). In spite of its popularity and widespread acceptance in clinical research, only recently has the reliability of the scale been addressed (Schag, et al. 1984). Our work and that of others suggest that the KPS is a reliable instrument; however, the absence of specific guidelines for its use has led to some modest inconsistency in ratings (Schag, et al. 1984).

The KPS as originally described is presented in Table 7.1. The scale ranges from 0 to 100 percent and is rated in deciles. For each subject completing the CIPS, the KPS was rated by the physician or a trained health professional who performed a structured interview (Schag, et al. 1984).

Table 7.1
Karnofsky Performance Status Scale

Condition	Percent	Comments
Able to carry on normal activity; no special care is needed	100%	Normal; no complaints, no evidence of disease
	90%	Able to carry on normal activity, minor signs or symptoms of disease
	80%	Normal activity with effort, some signs or symptoms of disease
Unable to work; able to live at home; cares for most personal needs; a varying amount of assistance is needed	70%	Cares for self; unable to carry on normal activity or to do active work
	60%	Requires occasional assistance but is able to care for most of own needs
	50%	Requires considerable assistance and frequent medical care
Unable to care for self; requires equivalent of institutional or hospital care; disease may be progressing rapidly	40%	Disabled; requires special medical care and assistance
	30%	Severely disabled; hospitalization is indicated, although death is not imminent.
	20%	Very sick; hospitalization is necessary; active supportive treatment necessary
	10%	Moribund; fatal processes progressing rapidly
	0%	Dead

Source: Compiled by the authors.

Subjects

The 320 subjects who form the sample for this review participated in our initial studies, between 1980 and 1982, which evaluated the psychometric properties of the CIPS (Schag, et al. 1983). Patients were recruited for these studies from several clinics at a large university cancer center (51.3%), a Veterans Administration Medical Center (32.5%), the private practice of two community oncologists (10%), and several other practice settings

(6.5%). Thus, the subjects came from a broad range of socioeconomic backgrounds. There were 238 men and 82 women in the sample. All subjects gave informed consent prior to participation in the study.

Analysis of Data

Descriptive statistics are used to examine data we have previously collected with the CIPS. Differences are assessed between working and nonworking subjects related to medical, socioeconomic, demographic, and functional performance status factors. The relationship between the cessation of work and its relationship to the time of cancer diagnosis is also examined. In addition, we describe responses to the CIPS in relation to work status.

MEDICAL AND DEMOGRAPHIC FINDINGS IN RELATION TO WORK

Summary of Results in 320 Cancer Patients

At the time the CIPS and associated instruments were completed, 94 subjects (29.4%) were working and 226 (70.6%) were not working. The percentage of subjects working at the time of this survey ranged from 43.3 percent at the University Medical Center to 6.7 percent at the VA Medical Center. There was an equal distribution of men and women according to work status. However, there was a significant difference in age between the working and nonworking subjects, with a mean age of 54.7 years for the working and a mean age of 59.9 years for the nonworking subjects (p = .000). There were no differences between the working and nonworking with regard to ethnicity or religion, but significantly more working subjects were married or in a significant relationship (81.9% versus 64.6%, p = .0033).

Major differences were found between the working and nonworking subjects regarding education, occupation, and KPS, which are presented in Tables 7.2, 7.3, and 7.4. Over 50 percent of the working subjects had a college level education or higher while only 21 percent of the nonworking subjects had attained this education level. Considerably more of the non-working subjects were in the lowest educational levels. There is a direct relationship between continued work and education level, with the highest rate of work among those in the highest educational level (Table 7.2). Few of the working subjects had blue-collar occupations, while nearly one-third of the nonworking subjects were in this group. Similarly, there is a direct relationship between higher occupation level and work (Table 7.3). The mean KPS for working subjects was significantly higher than for non-working subjects (90.7 versus 79.01, p = .000).

Table 7.2
Education and Work Status

Education Level	Working	Not Working	% Working/Level
College Level–Graduate or Professional School	48(51%)	57(21%)	45.7%
High School Graduate–Partial College	43(45.8%)	116(51.8%)	27%
Partial High School or less	3(3.2%)	63(27.2%)	4.5%
	94	226	

p=.000

Source: Compiled by the authors.

Table 7.3
Occupation and Work Status

Occupation Level	Working	Not Working	% Working/Level
1-2	28(29.7%)	25(11.1%)	52%
3-4	60(63.9%)	126(56%)	32%
5-7	6(6.5%)	75(32.9%)	7.5%
	94	226	

p=.000

1=Higher executive, proprietor, major professional

2=Business manager, proprietor of medium-sized business, lesser professional

3=Administrative person, owner small business, minor professional

4=Clerical and sales worker, technicians, owner of little business

5=Skilled manual work

6=Machine operators and semi-skilled

7=Unskilled, including homemakers, students and unemployed persons

Source: Compiled by the authors.

At the time of our survey, the median time since cancer diagnosis was the same for both working and nonworking subjects (13 months). However, the extent of disease at diagnosis was significantly different for the two groups (p = .0002). Seventy percent of the working subjects had limited and resectable disease at the time of diagnosis as compared to 44 percent of the nonworking subjects. The nonworking subjects had a higher incidence of metastatic disease at diagnosis (29.3%) than the working subjects (19.1%).

As a consequence, significantly more nonworking subjects had metastatic

Table 7.4
Karnofsky Performance Status and Work

KPS Level	Working	Not Working
80–100	95.7%	62.9%
50–70	4.3%	34%
0–40	0%	3.2%

p=.000

Source: Compiled by the authors.

Table 7.5
Cancer Site and Work Status★

Site	No. of Subjects	Working	Not Working
Breast	39	41%	59%
Colorectal	31	9.7%	90.3%
Lung	42	9.6%	90.4%
Lymphoma	15	20%	80%
Prostate	57	33.3%	66.7%
Renal	30	40%	60%
Testes	15	73%	27%
Transitional cell (GU)	38	50%	50%

★Selected, most common sites from sample of 320 subjects.

Source: Compiled by the authors.

disease at the time they completed the CIPS (49.8% of the nonworking versus 25.5% of the working subjects, p = .0001). Therefore, there were significant differences in the kind of treatments being received by each group at the time the CIPS was administered. Forty-four percent of the nonworking patients were receiving chemotherapy and 29.8 percent of the working were receiving chemotherapy (p = .0257). Fewer patients in both groups were receiving radiation therapy; however, more patients in the nonworking group were receiving this type of treatment (10.2% versus 1.1%, p = .0046).

Major differences in work status were observed in relation to specific cancer site and are described in Table 7.5. Only those sites with a significant number of subjects are listed and include cancers of the breast, colon, rectum, lung, prostate, kidneys, testes, urinary tract, and lymphomas. Relatively few (<10%) of the lung and colorectal cancer patients were working whereas over 70 percent of the testicular cancer patients continued to work.

The working and nonworking cancer patients also differed with regard to other medical characteristics. While the studies using the CIPS focused primarily on outpatients with cancer, all of the inpatients who participated in these studies were in the nonworking group and made up 11.6 percent of that sample. None of the working cancer patients were inpatients at the time of completing the CIPS (p = .0013). In addition, the nonworking group had a higher frequency of noncancer medical illnesses such as cardiac disease (p = .0014) and other medical conditions (p = .0066); however, there were no significant differences between the two groups in the frequency of diabetes or hypertension.

The relationship between the cessation of work and the time of cancer diagnosis was examined in the 222 nonworking subjects by using data from the background information form. This analysis demonstrated a close relationship between the cessation of work and the time of cancer diagnosis. Seventeen percent of the nonworking subjects had stopped work during the six months prior to their cancer diagnosis; 9.45 percent had stopped working at the time of their cancer diagnosis; an additional 23.8 percent discontinued work in the six months after diagnosis. Thus nearly 50 percent of the nonworking subjects stopped working in close temporal proximity to the diagnosis of cancer.

Analyses of Subgroups by KPS

Many of the medical differences between the working and nonworking subjects just described might be accounted for by differences in the KPS scores of the two groups. Therefore, we chose to examine two subgroups within the data set: all subjects with a KPS 80–100 and those with a KPS of 100. Patients with KPS scores of 80–100 have the functional ability to work (see Table 7.1). Since the KPS is rated in relationship to the patient's ability to work (Karnofsky, et al. 1949), we selected this variable to control for potential bias in the previous analyses.

Subgroup of Subjects with KPS 80–100

There were 90 working and 144 nonworking subjects in the subgroup of subjects with KPS 80–100. The mean KPS of the working subjects was 91.7 and for the nonworking subjects was 88.1 (p = .000). This suggests that even in this group the working patients had higher KPS scores. There was no difference in the distribution of men and women between the working and nonworking subjects. However, there was still a significant difference in the mean age of the two groups, but it was not as marked as in the total study sample (working: mean age 55.0 years, versus nonworking:

mean age 58.9 years, p = .019). There were no differences between the two groups in relation to religion or ethnicity. The same pattern of marital status persisted in this subgroup of patients as in the larger sample, that is, a significantly greater number of the working subjects were in a marital or similar relationship.

Significant differences were found between the working and nonworking subjects with respect to occupation and education. The pattern of the distributions (occupation and education) were identical to the larger study population and the frequency of work according to cancer site was similar to the larger study population. Other medical characteristics, such as time since cancer diagnosis, extent of disease at diagnosis, presence of metastases, and pattern of other medical illnesses, were similar to the larger sample; however, in contrast to the larger sample, fewer of the nonworking subjects had metastatic disease at the time they completed the CIPS (37.1% vs. 49.8% in the larger sample). Similar to the larger sample, nearly 50 percent of those patients who were not working had discontinued work during the six months preceding, at, or following the diagnosis of cancer.

Subgroup of Subjects with KPS 100

Since there were still significant differences in the mean KPS rating of the subgroup of patients with KPS 80–100, we were concerned that the other differences might be related to KPS. The subgroup of patients with a KPS of 100 represents the most homogeneous and the most healthy subgroup. The same analyses were conducted on this group since there should be no identifiable functional cause for not working. Analysis of this subgroup was performed to identify significant demographic or medical variables that could influence the individual's work status. There were 31 working and 23 nonworking subjects with a KPS of 100. There was a significant difference in age between the working and nonworking subjects (51.5 years versus 62 years, p = .003), which is more marked than similar comparisons in the preceding analyses. In contrast to the whole sample and the KPS 80–100 subgroup, there were no differences between the working and nonworking subjects in relation to extent of disease at diagnosis, current care status, occupation, education, or marital status. As in the larger samples, there was an even distribution of women, and there were no differences in religion or ethnicity. Thus, these nonworking and working subjects differed significantly only in age, with the means being more than a decade apart.

None of the subjects with KPS 100 were receiving chemotherapy, and one subject who was working was receiving radiation therapy. Only one subject had metastatic disease, and this individual was in the nonworking group. There were no differences between the working and nonworking subjects with KPS 100 related to cancer site. The distribution of cancer sites

Table 7.6
Cancer Site and Work Status in Subjects with KPS 100

Site	No. of Subjects	Working	Not Working
Breast	6	66.7%	33.3%
Colorectal	6	50%	50%
Gastric	1	0%	100%
Head/Neck	1	100%	0%
Hodgkins	2	50%	50%
Lung	1	0%	100%
Lymphoma	3	0%	100%
Prostate	9	55.6%	44.4%
Renal	5	60%	40%
Testes	7	85.7%	14.3%
Transitional cell (GU)	10	60%	40%
Misc.	2	50%	50%

Source: Compiled by the authors.

in this subgroup is presented in Table 7.6. The only medical characteristic that was significantly different between the working and nonworking subjects was a higher frequency of other medical illnesses in the nonworking subjects (p = .0014). In contrast to the larger samples, less than 30 percent of these nonworking subjects had discontinued work in close temporal relation (six months before or after diagnosis) to the cancer diagnosis, with more than 40 percent having stopped work more than a year before the cancer diagnosis.

In summary, the working and nonworking subjects with KPS 100 are distinguishable primarily by age and frequency of other medical illnesses. The nonworking subjects are older, have more chronic disease, and have stopped working more than a year before their cancer diagnosis, suggesting that the cessation of work was independent of the symptoms or problems related to cancer diagnosis and treatment.

FINDINGS FROM THE CIPS

The CIPS contains several specific problem statements that relate to work. Two items relate to the individuals' ability to hold a full-time or part-time job. There were significant differences in the responses of the subjects to these two questions based on their current work status (p = .000). The 94

Table 7.7

Responses to the CIPS Work Questions in 94 Working Subjects

QUESTION	NOT AT ALL A PROBLEM	MILD TO MODERATE PROBLEM	SEVERE PROBLEM
Difficulty talking to boss	83%	10.6%	6.4%
Communication with people at work	74.5%	15.9%	9.6%
Difficulty telling boss I can't do things	81.9%	11.7%	6.4%
Difficulty asking for time off for treatments	89.4%	6.4%	4.3%
Difficulty finding a new job	91.5%	2.2%	6.4%
Problems working full-time job	78.7%	13.8%	7.5%
Problems working part-time job	94.7%	3.2%	2.2%

Source: Compiled by the authors.

working subjects all responded to these two questions and five additional questions which relate to communication at work and job seeking. Their responses are described in Table 7.7. The responses to these specific CIPS items reveal that most patients are having minimal difficulties in the work place. However, there are problems with communication at work for approximately 25 percent of the subjects (range 25.5% for communication with people at work to 10.6% for asking for time off from work for treatments). We did not specifically ask our respondents whether or not they were working full- or part-time; nevertheless, it is of interest that 21.3 percent of those who were working reported that the cancer or its treatment caused problems with working a full-time job. Fewer subjects reported problems with working a part-time job.

The CIPS examines a broad range of daily activities not specifically related to work; nevertheless, problems with many of these activities may affect the cancer patient's ability to work. The CIPS is divided into 22 scales which relate to specific areas of daily living. Our previous work has shown that patients with more extensive disease and lower KPS scores have more problems reflected on their CIPS responses. A review of these scale scores in the working and nonworking subjects was made for the entire sample of 320 subjects, for those subjects with KPS 80–100, and for subjects with KPS 100. The nonworking subjects had significantly more problems in a wide range of areas, with the most differences noted in the large sample and the fewest differences in the KPS 100 subgroup. These factor scale score differences are presented in Table 7.8.

The whole sample contains a large number of nonworking subjects with significantly poorer KPS scores, thus accounting for the wide range of differences in a number of the factor scales, especially worry, clothing, body image, and interaction with family and friends. There are a number of differences that persist in the KPS 80–100 group and these are more interesting. They include problems with functional health status, such as bending, lifting, self-care and fatigue; cognitive difficulties; weight maintenance; and communication with friends and relatives. Difficulty working is also a significant problem area for the nonworking subjects with KPS 80–100. Lastly, there are very few differences in the factor scale scores between the working and nonworking subjects in the KPS 100 subgroup; however, it is of interest that these nonworking subjects report significantly more problems in the areas of functional health status. This most likely relates to the older age of the nonworking subjects as well as the higher frequency of other noncancer medical illnesses described earlier for this subgroup of nonworking subjects. The only additional scale score difference between KPS 100 working and nonworking subjects was in the area of control of the medical staff.

DISCUSSION AND CONCLUSIONS

This cross-sectional study of 320 cancer patients uses the CIPS and associated instruments to examine the relationship between work status and a variety of medical, demographic, and socioeconomic factors. This study validates previous demographic and socioeconomic observations about work and cancer. Patients with a higher socioeconomic status (education and occupation status) more frequently work than those who have a lower socioeconomic status (Feldman 1976, 1978; Greenleigh 1979). Those individuals who are younger are more likely to continue working than those who are older (Feldman 1976, 1978, 1980; Greenleigh 1979). In addition, the ability to work with a diagnosis of cancer varies by specific cancer site (Greenleigh 1979; Mellette 1985). Some new observations from this review are that working subjects are more likely to be married (or in a significant

Table 7.8
CIPS Factor Scale Score Difference for Working versus Nonworking
Subjects by Analysis Group

Scale	Whole Sample	KPS 80 – 100	KPS 100
Communication with M.D.	p=.001	p=.03	----
Chemotherapy problems	---	---	---
Functional health status	p=.000	p=.000	p=.001
Worry	p=.029	---	---
Cognitive difficulties	p=.000	p=.044	---
Obtaining information from health care team	p=.002	p=.008	---
Body Image	p=.022	------	---
Weight maintenance	p=.000	p=.000	---
Communication with friends and relatives	p=.000	p=.013	---
Compliance	------	-------	---
Clothing	p=.022	-------	---
Control of medical staff	------	--------	p=.048
Discomfort with procedures	-----	-------	---
Difficulty working	p=.000	p=.000	---
Difficulty inter- acting with family and friends	p=.001	-------	---

Scale	Whole Sample	KPS 80 – 100	KPS 100
Anxiety in medical situations	——————	———————	———
Communication with partner	——————	———————	———
Affection with partner	——————	————————	———
Sexual dysfunction	———————	-———————	———
Interaction with partner	——————	————————	———
Sex Interest	——————	————————	———
Care by partner	——————	————————	———

Source: Compiled by the authors.

relationship) than nonworking subjects, and among those subjects who do not continue to work after a cancer diagnosis, a large percentage discontinue work within the six months preceding or following their cancer diagnosis.

In this study we have characterized some of the medical factors that are associated with nonworking status among cancer patients. These include more extensive disease at diagnosis, current metastatic disease, current treatment with chemotherapy, and other noncancer medical illnesses. Nonworking cancer patients who have a KPS of 80–100, which should predict the capability of working, have more problems with cognitive function, functional health status, and weight maintenance (see Table 7.8), all of which may have a negative impact on the ability to work (Silberfarb, 1983).

In our sample of 94 working cancer patients, surprisingly few serious problems were identified in relationship to communication at work, although 25 percent of the subjects did describe some problems with communication with colleagues at work. Problems working a full-time job were also of concern to over 20 percent of these subjects, suggesting the possibility of problems with job performance.

Our current research with the CIPS includes more specific and detailed information about the cancer patient's current work status, recent changes in employment, as well as desire to return to work if currently unemployed. Future analyses should give us more accurate information about the interaction of cancer and work. The ability to return to work after a cancer diagnosis is influenced by a variety of factors, many of which interact independently with one another, including previous education level, previous occupation, employment status immediately preceding the cancer diagnosis, specific cancer site, and extent of disease at diagnosis. Some of these factors are also interrelated, such as cancer site, and socioeconomic status and occupational level, so that some individuals may have several factors that impact negatively on the likelihood of continued work after a cancer diagnosis. Age seems to be a separate and important factor that influences work status in cancer patients (Greenleigh 1979).

From this review we have observed that the working cancer patient is more likely to be married, younger in age, and have a higher educational and occupational level. In addition, the working patient usually had resectable or limited disease at diagnosis and is less likely to be receiving chemotherapy for metastatic disease while working. Cancer site also plays an important role in the ability to work. Many breast, genitourinary, and prostate cancer patients continue to work while few patients with lung and colorectal cancer are working.

REFERENCES

Berry, W. R., Laszlo, J., Cox, E., et al. Prognostic factors in metastatic and hormally unresponsive carcinoma of the prostate. *Cancer*, 1979, *44*, 763–775.

Feldman, F. L. *Work and cancer health histories: A study of the experience of recovered patients.* San Francisco: American Cancer Society, California Division, 1976.

Feldman, F. L. *Work and cancer health histories: A study of the experiences of recovered blue-collar workers.* Oakland: American Cancer Society, California Division, 1978.

Feldman, F. L. *Work and cancer health histories: Work expectations and experiences of youth with cancer histories.* Oakland: American Cancer Society, California Division, 1980.

Greenleigh Associates, Inc. *Report on the social, economic and psychological needs of cancer patients in California.* Oakland: American Cancer Society, California Division, 1979.

Heinrich, R. L., Schag, C. C., & Ganz, P. A. Living with cancer: The cancer inventory of problem situations. *Journal of Clinical Psychology*, 1984, *2*, 187–193.

Karnofsky, D. A., & Burchenal, J. H. The clinical evaluation of chemotherapeutic agents in cancer. In C. M. Macleod (Ed.), *Evaluation of chemotherapeutic agents.* New York: Columbia University Press, 1949, 199–205.

Mellette, S. J. The cancer patient at work. *Ca—A Cancer Journal for Clinicians*, 1985, *35*, 360–373.

Schag, C. C., Heinrich, R. L., & Ganz, P. A. Karnofsky performance status revisited: Reliability, validity and guidelines. *Journal of Clinical Oncology*, 1984, *2*, 187–193.

Schag, C. C., Heinrich, R. L., & Ganz, P. A. Cancer inventory of problem situations: An instrument for assessing cancer patients' rehabilitation needs. *Journal of Psychosocial Oncology* 1983, *1*, 11–24.

Silverfarb, P. M. Chemotherapy and cognitive deficits in cancer patients. *Annual Review of Medicine*, 1983, *34*, 35–46.

Stanley, K. E. Prognostic factors for survival in patients with inoperable lung cancer. *Journal of the National Cancer Institute*, 1980, *65*, 25–32.

II

Conclusions

8

Maximizing the Productive Activities of the Cancer Patient: Research Issues

Ivan Barofsky

INTRODUCTION

The data presented in this volume, and available in the literature (Mellette & Franco 1987), have revealed several consistent findings. First, the childhood cancer patient's work history is significantly, and adversely, affected by their having had and been treated for cancer (Feldman; Holmes, et al; and Teta, this volume). These adverse effects can be illustrated by the increased number of reports of less than adequate insurance coverage; until recently, total rejection from the military; disruption and limitation of career objectives; and the large proportion of patients that deny the existence of their disease to prospective employers. These outcomes have been labeled discriminatory, in that the person's disease has become part of the events associated with decisions concerning their work and personal history, whereas they would not have if the person did not have cancer.

The impact of cancer on the person with an established work history is less clear, although it has been found that a majority of persons treated with cancer return to work. The percentage returning to work varies as a function of age, sex, type of employment, size of employer, disease severity, and disease, among other factors. Thus, Feldman's (1978) original observation that the percentage of blue-collar workers who do not return to work is considerably higher than white-collar workers has been replicated (Ganz, et al., this volume). Feldman's work suggests that employment problems are determined by employers' attitudes and preferences, the wage and benefits available as a function of occupational status, and related issues—factors

that are external to the individual and can be labeled evidence of job discrimination. In contrast, Houts, et al. (this volume), finds that persons
reporting employment problems are younger, have sought professional help
for emotional problems prior to diagnosis, have received chemotherapy,
and have an advanced stage of the disease at diagnosis. The Houts, et al.,
data suggest that reports of work problems by cancer patients are more a
function of the individual's disease and psychological status, than of the
economic system or organizational dynamic within which he or she is
employed. Fobair's et al. (this volume), data bridge the gap between these
alternative views. Using Heilman's Lack-of-Fit model, Fobair, et al. (Table
6.6; this volume), found that of the 64 percent of the persons who reported
problems with their work, two-thirds of these problems involved negative
evaluations of others, and only a third involved negative self-evaluation.
Although Fobair's data are self-reports, they do suggest that factors both
external and internal to the individual may determine the work history of
the cancer patient.

The studies referred to above are consistent in that they represent retrospective or outcome studies of an extremely dynamic and interactive
process. Outcome studies, by their very nature, may fail to reveal differences
in the processes that lead to what may even be the same outcome. This
makes selection of a control group, and the study of work history processes,
critical future research issues—issues best addressed in the context of a
prospective study of the impact of cancer on work history.

Some of the reported studies (Mellette & Franco 1987) have included
comparison groups (e.g., Houts, et al.; and Teta, this volume, both used
sibling controls), but most have not. Most studies represent convenience
samples, although the Houts, et al. (this volume), study does permit population-based estimates. The Houts, et al., study is limited, however, in
that the work history data were collected retrospectively and were based
on a limited number of questions embedded in a needs assessment questionnaire. Thus, the requirement for process-oriented prospective studies
with appropriate control groups leaves ample opportunity for the conduct
of innovative research.

The Impact of Cancer on the Person with an Established Work History

Cancer is a disease that predominantly strikes persons 50 years old and
older (Cancer Statistics 1988), a good proportion of whom may be working
at disease onset. Thus, the largest sample of persons with cancer will already
have an established work history, or pattern of productive activities. For
these patients determining the impact of cancer represents the detection of
a change against a background of change. Thus, work, housekeeping, and
being a student each has a natural history and cancer may speed up the
sequence of events (as happens with persons who retire early), slow it down

Table 8.1
Work and Cancer: A Research Agenda

1. THE IMPACT OF CANCER ON THE PERSON WITH AN ESTABLISHED WORK HISTORY.

a. Changes in the Wages and Benefits of the Employed Patient
b. Health Insurance Costs of the Cancer Patient
c. Work Transitions: Job Establishment and Termination
d. Job Dynamics
e. Impact on Other Forms of Productive Activities

2. THE CHILDHOOD CANCER SURVIVOR AND WORK HISTORY

a. Occupational Choice
b. Occupational Competence

3. WORK-ABLENESS

a. Physical Assessments
b. Performance Appraisals
c. Worker-to-job Fit

4. STUDIES OF JOB DISCRIMINATION

a. Economic Models of Employment Discrimination.
b. Social Psychological Aspects of Employment Discrimination.

5. ELEMENTS OF A INTERVENTION PROGRAM

a. The Epidemiology of Work Adjustment
b. Design Issues
c. Statistical Issues

6. SUMMARY

Source: Compiled by author.

(as when the person stays in a job, rather than risk career progression that might jeopardize the availability of health insurance, or drops out of school before graduation), or diversify it into other forms of productive activity (as when the person assumes voluntary activities instead of working for a living). Knowing this, the following studies are proposed in Table 8.1.

Studies of Changes in the Fiscal Status (as Measured by Changes in Wages and Benefits) of the Employed Patient

There have only been a limited number of purely economic studies of the fiscal consequences of cancer. Most of these studies are based on secondary analyses of financial data or retrospective patient and psychological processing. These studies would not only be useful as part of cost-effectiveness analyses but also provide a data base to compare to perceived changes in wages and benefits.

Studies of the Health Insurance Costs of the Cancer Patient

Is it true that the cost of cancer care leads to an increase in a group's health or life insurance costs? How much does it cost the insurance companies to pay for the cost of cancer care? Is the increase in a group rate more likely due to the inflation of medical care or the cost of catastrophic, but low frequency events, such as cancer care? What is the comparative cost of care of major illnesses? Is the cost of cancer care significantly greater than that of other chronic diseases? What are the differences in cost between types of cancer?

The answers to the above questions are important since there is a widespread belief that cancer care disproportionately increases the cost of group rates, justifying discriminatory practices. The answers to these research questions are also relevant to the childhood cancer survivor.

Studies of Work Transitions: Job Establishment and Termination

Getting a job and leaving a job have to be two of the more complex human experiences. Yet, there has been a minimum of cancer-related research in this area. One approach to the research task is to derive testable hypotheses from theoretical statements. Parkes' paper (1971) describing the consequences of changes in status of a person as a result of *psychosocial transitions*, provides one such theoretical statement. Parkes (1971, p. 103) sees psychosocial transitions as "those major changes in life space that are lasting in their effects, which take place over a relatively short period of time and which affect large areas of the assumptive world." Life space refers to the world within which the individual acts and interacts, while the assumptive world refers to the assumptions the person holds about how his or her world works. During psychosocial transitions the life space and assumptive world of the person may both change in a dynamic and interactive manner. Parkes' conceptual framework has been elaborated on for the unemployed (Hayes & Nutman 1981), but has also been used to account for the psychological consequences of cancer (Parkes 1975; Mages & Mendelsohn 1979).

Table 8.2 summarizes the sequence of transitions associated with a person's psychosocial response to chronic unemployment and the medical transitions of the cancer patient. What is striking is the similarity in the emotional responses to the two different experiences. For example, it is not uncommon for patients to delay seeking medical advice when they first discover what may be a sign of illness, much as the unemployed initially become immobilized after discovering they have lost their jobs. Cancer patients usually talk about "beating" cancer during the initial treatment phase of their illness and thereby try to minimize the psychological impact of the events happening to them, not unlike the unemployed person who attempts to find a job. As the damage to one's body becomes evident for the cancer patient, and the inability to find a job becomes evident to the unemployed, both may become depressed. Finally, both may have to accept the permanent nature of the changes in their lives, and accommodate themselves to a new reality.

Table 8.2
Transitions

MEDICAL TRANSITIONS OF THE CANCER PATIENT	PSYCHOSOCIAL TRANSITIONS OF THE CHRONICALLY UMEMPLOYED
1. Discovery of Symptoms; Being Diagnosed	1. Immobilization; Learning of Job Loss
2. Primary Treatment; "Fight Cancer"	2. Minimization; Seek Job
3. Damage to One's Body; Depression	3. Loss of Confidence; Depression
4. Maintaining Continuity	4. Acceptance of Reality-Letting Go
5. Possibility of Recurrence	5. Testing
6. Persistent or Recurrent Disease	6. Search for Meaning
7. Terminal Illness; Acceptance	7. Internalization; Acceptance

Source: Compiled by author.

Without forcing the parallels between the two transition processes, their similarity does generate a number of interesting hypotheses to test. First, the fact that the psychosocial transitions that the cancer patient is experiencing are similar to what the unemployed person experiences suggests that a considerable portion of the variance associated with psychosocial responses to cancer may be psychosocial responses to unemployment. Testing this hypothesis would involve comparing the distress created by losing one's job to someone's developing cancer. A moderate correlation would be expected, especially since it is known that when health issues become evident they displace the previous primary concerns (such as work and income) of most individuals (Bergermaier, et al. 1984). Thus, a reorganization of the value structure of an individual occurs with the acceptance of being a cancer patient (one's life is threatened) that may confound demonstrating that the distress associated with loss of a job, or inability to return to work, of the cancer patient is contributing to current distress. Still, the magnitude if not the quality of the distress may be similar for the two study groups, although the context for persons judging their distress may be quite different.

This suggests a second hypothesis to test, which is whether or not the sequence of emotional responses is similar for the two experiences.

A third hypothesis that grows from the previous two is whether returning to work or continuing to work during their treatment will minimize the distress cancer patients experience. This type of study is also not simple, because a person may lose his or her job but find meaning in life by becoming involved in other forms of productive activities, or may accept as real the argument that he or she has the right to retire early, or reorganize life since the duration of the life has now been questioned. Thus, while complex, it would seem very important to determine the extent work transitions contribute to the distress and psychosocial responses of the cancer patient.

Job Dynamics

There has never been a systematic study of the impact of cancer on job dynamics. What is known about the contribution of job dynamics to job discrimination is limited to retrospective self-reports by the affected worker and rarely by co-workers.

Job dynamics refers to the interpersonal relationship between persons engaged in a common occupational activity. As Salaman (1986) states, job dynamics are patterned, such that the frequency, intimacy, and significance of contacts are not distributed equally. Freedman (1984) states that the function of job interactions is to minimize risk, and to develop a shelter from market-based job insecurities (much as unions provide for workers). Thus, one research question that can be asked is whether cancer, or changes in the physical status of the patient, can become one of the criteria in the formal and informal group formations that occur in the workplace.

Since most work patterns are established by the time a worker develops cancer, an equally relevant issue is how membership in work groups influences the decision-making activities of the patient. Do such groups become a social support system for cancer patients, sustaining them in their efforts or do these groups convince persons to retire early, work part-time, etc.? It would be of particular interest to determine if some of this influence can be interpreted as self-serving, whereby convincing a person with cancer to retire the group reduces their own "market-based job insecurities," to use Freedman's phrase (1984).

One of the determinants of job dynamics is job organization. Varying the extent a worker can be a craftsman, or is required to do repetitive tasks will determine the work context and, therefore, the nature and extent of co-worker interaction. Since job organization will affect productivity, it has also become a significant determinant of job dynamics. Thus, the breaking up of a job into components and having these components performed by different workers, the so-called de-skilling of jobs, illustrates how job organization can determine productivity, and indirectly job dynamics. Taylorism, or the Scientific Management of Work, provides a theoretical rationale for this effort (Littler 1982).

Job organization, as a structural determinant of job dynamics, may help account for the observation that blue-collar workers with cancer experience more job discrimination than white-collar workers with cancer. Blue-collar workers may experience more discrimination because their jobs are de-skilled, broken into component parts so that only one part of the work task is performed by an individual worker. Replacement of this worker is relatively easy when compared to replacing a professional who is more integrated into a work organization, and whose loss would have a greater chance of impacting productivity. A direct test of this hypothesis, however, would require being able to gauge the "replaceability" of the job of the person with cancer, which may be a research task unto itself.

Impact on Other Forms of Productive Activities

Houseworkers, students, and retirees also develop cancer and they also reorganize how they spend their time. Of particular interest, and not yet the focus of any deliberate study, is whether the impact of cancer moves an individual along a hierarchy of productive activities. Thus, a worker may decide to take some courses or help out more with the housework, or a houseworker may decide to do voluntary work, or increase his or her recreational reading.

Also of interest is at what point the proportion of nonproductive activities exceeds productive activities. Is there a high degree of relationship between nonproductive activities and terminal illness? Is it possible that the terminally ill who maintain a high proportion of productive activities have a higher sense of well-being? Statistical procedures, such as path analysis and stochastic modeling (see, e.g., Diekmann & Mitter 1984), would be very helpful in mathematically describing these processes.

A complementary study that avoids the prejudgment of activities as being productive or not would involve determining if the person with cancer has reorganized his or her value structure. The presence of such a reorganization would then help account for changes in activities.

The Cancer Survivor and Work History

Many of the studies proposed above will include, as subjects, childhood cancer survivors. Thus, the studies to be proposed in this section need only deal with issues unique to the development of a personal work history. This includes the person with cancer choosing an occupation and then becoming occupationally competent.

The evidence that the childhood cancer survivor's occupational career is adversely affected by illness is evident from several sources of data (c.f., Mellette & Franco 1986). Teta (Chapter 3, this volume) found, for example, that males, as compared to their brothers, did not do as well occupationally. Occupational status was measured by whether they were ever employed; level of income, if employed; and job skill level and tenure in job. In contrast, female survivors overall did better than male survivors but did reveal deficits, when compared to their sisters, in job tenure and skill level. These effects occurred even though the survivors' educational achievements were comparable to their siblings. These outcomes could not be attributed to brain tumor survivors, the treatment of which (by radiotherapy or chemotherapy directly to the brain) may impact the intellectural capacity (Brouwers, et al. 1985) and, therefore, occupational achievement of the patients.

Phillips, et al. (1985), in a study of 83 childhood leukemia survivors, found that the parents of the survivors had higher occupational status than their children, although the children's status was comparable to what would be expected for the population as a whole.

These studies suggest that understanding process variables, such as how the cancer survivor selects a career and how he or she becomes competent in the selected occupation, would be important when trying to account for such outcome measures as job tenure, skill level, and so on.

Occupational Choice

What career does a childhood cancer survivor select? How, if in any way, are such decisions affected by being treated for and surviving cancer? That occupational choice is an important issue in work history has been amply demonstrated for the general population (Barofsky [Chapter 1], this volume), but little is known concerning such choices for the chronically ill, such as the childhood cancer survivor. Prospective, longitudinal studies of the factors that determine occupational decision making by childhood cancer survivors are required to clarify the answers to the above questions.

Occupational Competence

Determining the occupational competence of the childhood cancer survivor is proposed to be a major research objective. The reason for this is straightforward. Occupational competence is of importance because it is one measure of the degree to which an individual has realized his or her potential, and maximizing the potential of the cancer survivor has to be one of the basic rationales for interest in this area of research.

Occupational competence may be defined as a measure of the *effectiveness* of the job-related behaviors, coping skills (e.g., how well the individual responds to changes in job requirements), or problem-solving abilities required to function in a wide range of occupational contexts. Occupational competence may be studied as either a process (how competence develops), or outcome (level of competence achieved) measure, or reflect a level of occupational activity (such as the point to which a person has progressed in a career development track). Occupational competence deals with a subset of issues that includes interpersonal and social competencies, but is confined to work-related activities.

The occupational competence approach to work-related activities avoids the pitfalls of labeling persons as defective and instead emphasizes the development of competence, and when deficient, assists people in becoming more effective in managing problems related to work. Many individuals with limitations in functioning are still able to maximize particular domains of their activities. Thus, Zubin and Spring (1977) found that schizophrenics may still have work competence before, after, or even during hospitalization for a psychotic episode. The data are similar for the person who develops cancer with an established work history; some patients continuing to work during and after treatment for cancer. The problem is different for the childhood cancer survivor who has to become occupationally competent in the presence of the consequence of a disease, and/or its treatment, and it is this process which would be the focus of the proposed research.

Confounding any study of occupational competence is the fact that administrative or organizational issues can determine the career outcome, independent of any individual imput, of a childhood cancer survivor. For example, administrative or organizational issues can confound the development of occupational competence by either under- or over-utilizing the skills of the person. O'Brien, et al. (1978), surveyed 1381 employees and found that approximately a third reported that their jobs under-utilized their skills, while a third over-utilized their skills.

Self-reports, which was what the O'Brien, et al. (1978), report was based on, can also be distorted by the expectations of the worker. The literature (O'Brien 1986) suggests that there are two "objective" approaches to the measurement of under-utilization. The first matches the level of education of the employee to that required by the job, while the second looks at the de-skilling of jobs. Thus, using observers who are independent of the situation, it should be possible to judge if childhood cancer patients' jobs under-utilize their skills.

The longitudinal studies that would be most advantageous to perform to study these issues seriously requires a level and persistence of commitment, both fiscal and intellectual, that few institutions can mount. Large corporations may be willing to make such a commitment but would, by their nature, limit the range of experiences of the cancer patients. A prototype of an appropriate type of study is the AT&T longitudinal study of managers (Bray & Howard 1983). It is limited, however, in that it only deals with managers in a company known for its responsiveness to individual worker needs. An alternative approach would use newly diagnosed patients identified through a tumor registry or tertiary care center who would then be followed for an extended period of time.

Work-ableness

The cancer patient, like many persons with chronic diseases, can experience a wide range of functional outcomes following treatments. A reasonably large proportion of the patients show no long-term consequences of their treatment, while some will be disabled with manifest limitations of function. The exact proportions of each are not known. What is known, at least for patients with chronic illnesses, is that as improved treatments and earlier detection lead to decreased mortality, there will be a correlated increase in the number of persons with limitations in work ability (J. J. Feldman 1982). Thus, the more likely that a patient survive cancer the more likely it will be that he or she will have some impairment of his or her work capacity.

One of the critical questions asked by employers is whether recovered cancer patients are able to continue their work at the level they engaged in prior to treatment for their disease. Employers want to know the answer to this question for humanitarian reasons, but also to ensure themselves that the continued employment of the patient will not adversely affect productivity. Employers are also interested in knowing whether their employees with cancer are malingering, and, if not disabled, how long they will remain able. An employer's implicit or explicit answers to these questions become part of the decisions that can eventuate in a discriminatory act.

Work-ableness, its legal and empirical basis, has an extensive history, since it it relevant to all types of cases dealing with employment discrimination. For example, there is a considerable case record dealing with court rulings on weight-lifting restrictions and height and weight requirements of jobs (Hogan & Quigley 1986). What is usually litigated in these cases is whether the job requirement is necessary for performance of the job. This process can be illustrated when employers defend themselves against sex discrimination cases. What an employer has to do is prove that there is a bona fide occupational qualification associated with the job. To do this he or she must show that gender is related to job performance, is "necessary" for successful job performance, and that the job performance is a major determinant of the employer's business (Hogan & Quigley 1986). A bathroom attendant is an example of a job for which gender is a bona fide occupational qualification.

Pressure for the physical assessment of the cancer patient will increase not only because the absolute number of cancer patients with physical limitations will increase, but also because employers are increasingly going to want to defend themselves against litigation when they feel obligated to terminate an employee who has cancer. In addition, it will be important to understand the relationship between physical capacity and performance. One of the tactics that can be used to resolve differences between the physical requirements of a job and the performance of a patient is to maximize the fit of a worker to his or her job. Each of these topics will be discussed below.

Physical Assessment

The basic objective of a physical or medical assessment should be to ensure that a hiring procedure not discriminate against a functionally limited or disabled person and that a productive and qualified person be selected for a job. There are two basic types of physical assessment: a medical assessment and a job specific assessment.

A medical assessment usually consists of a physical examination and/or certification that the employee is capable of engaging in the normal range of activities associated with working. It seldom includes tests that are job specific. It uses a person's past or current medical history to evaluate his or her work-ableness, suitability for life insurance, and so on. In this approach medical diagnoses are used to screen out ineligible, not select eligible, applicants.

Job specific assessments usually involve formal physical ability testing, with all of the associated questions involving the reliability and validity of any standardized test. A standardized weight-lifting test for firemen might be a prototype of such a test. The consensus of those who specialize in employment discrimination law seems to be that the probability of legally substantiating that a physical abilities test when applied to an individual is valid, is slight (Koral 1980; Scott 1977). This is so because a job analysis, the initial step in an ability test construction procedure, varies as a function of the method used; the content of a test is usually a convenience sample and not representative of a behavioral or physical domain, and if representative of the population as a whole, not reflective of a minority group, disabled group, or other such. Notwithstanding these limitations, job specific assessments are commonly used selection devices.

An alternative to a screening and/or normative selection approach is the "Individual Assessment Hiring Procedure" (IAHP) proposed by the Medical Standards Project (1983, a joint effort of the California-based Disability Rights and Educational Defense Fund, the Employment Law Center of the Legal Aid Society of San Francisco, and an Advisory Committee of disability experts). The IAHP provides an employer with a set of procedures that are designed to individualize but yet answer a relevant set of questions when deciding to employ a functionally limited or disabled applicant (see Table 8.3).

The first three questions in the IAHP mandate that a job analysis be performed. The job analysis in this context differs from one used to develop a job selection test, since its intent is to analyze a job a particular person performs rather than analyze a job that may be performed by a variety of persons in a variety of contexts. The purpose of the job analysis is to ensure that nonjob-related physical conditions or disabilities are not used to disqualify an applicant; to determine if reasonable accommodations can be made to enable a disabled applicant to perform safely and efficiently; to protect the employee with limitations in function from further injury through accommodation or transfer; and to justify, both to the employee and the employer, finding alternative jobs for the employee and thereby minimizing pension, disability, retirement, and workmen's compensation costs.

Table 8.3
The Individual Assessment Hiring Procedure

1. What are the duties of the particular position in question?

2. What are the essential duties of the position?

3. What is physically required for the safe and efficient performance of the essential duties of the position?

4. Is the individual applicant currently able to physically perform all of the essential duties of the position safely and efficiently?

5. If not, is there any accommodation which, if provided, would enable the applicant to so perform?

6. If so, would the provision of this accommodation impose an undue hardship on the employer?

Source: Medical Standards Project, 1983.

The IAHP procedure recommends that if a person is currently qualified for the job that he or she be offered the job contingent upon a successful *pre-placement* physical examination. Thus, instead of making a job offer contingent upon a successful physical examination the IAHP makes *continued employment* dependent on demonstrated fitness. This procedural difference permits the employer to avoid charges of engaging in a discriminatory act, yet provides a way to avoid employing persons who have limitations of function, or disabilities that can have an adverse impact on productivity or lead to excessive costs for accommodation. It also gives the employee an opportunity to show that he or she has been able to compensate for what appears as a limitation in function or a frank disability, prior to a critical decision being made about continued employability.

An equitable evaluation process will require that the pre-placement medical examination be carefully considered: who does it, when should it be given, and who is told about the results of the examination. The evaluation process helps an employer evaluate an employee's current qualifications, not future risk. In general, the courts and legal precedent may have to be consulted for an employer to proceed with confidence when using future risk as a basis for evaluation.

The final phase of the hiring process involves determining if the applicant can perform all essential duties of the position safely and efficiently; if not, whether accommodation is possible; and if accommodation is required, whether it would impose an undue hardship on the employer. The Medical Standards Project (1983) recommends that the final hiring decision be made as a team effort, involving all personnel that are relevant to the task (e.g., personnel officer, supervisor, affirmative action officers, examining physician, etc.). It also recommends that an appeals mechanism be established for disqualified applicants.

Basically what the IAHP does is to insist that a physical assessment become part of a larger process, and that this process govern how an employer proceeds to make decisions concerning the employability of an applicant. It represents a viable alternative to the mechanical application of screening and job selection procedures, although the cost-effectiveness of each procedure remains an important research question.

The most obvious research problem is to determine the proportion of cancer patients who have physical limitations and to determine if this proportion is different from what is found for the population as a whole, or for persons with other types of chronic diseases. What is the relationship between physical limitations and type and stage of cancer? It might be particularly important to know how often a patient's physical limitations impact their work performance.

Also of interest, is whether it is possible to scale different types of limitations of function or disabilities along a common dimension. What would this dimension be, and can the scaled items be used to quantitate the outcome of a physical assessment? An effort like this would be limited by the fact that the context within which a disability is being expressed may determine its impact on the work-ableness of the patient. For example, a desk job is not necessarily adversely affected if the person has a lower extremity amputation, but there are many other types of jobs that would be.

Performance Appraisals

The complexity of a performance appraisal was discussed in Chapter 1 (Barofsky, this volume; see also, Berk 1986). The first question that has to be asked here is whether there is or is not a problem. Self-reports by patients do not provide much evidence of an adverse impact of cancer and its treatments on job performance (see, e.g., Fobair, et al.; Houts, et al., this volume). These data, however, may underestimate the magnitude of the problem since the effects may be subtle and be confounded by the capacity of individuals to adapt, as occurs in response to age-related changes in performance. Available studies have also been uniformly retrospective in nature. The anthropological-sociological method of using work diaries to collect intimate and detailed data concerning the immediate experiences of a person is not a frequently used research tool in studies of the work history of the cancer patient.

Cancer and its treatments may have a direct or indirect effect on job performance. Direct effects differ from indirect effects in that it is more likely that a physical impact, or biological change can be demonstrated, whereas indirect effects may be more reactive, and therefore psychological in nature. In most situations both direct and indirect effects will be involved. Impaired cognitive functioning (as occurs following prophylactic radiotherapy to the brain) or peripheral neuropathies (which result from some forms of chemotherapy) would be considered examples of direct effects.

Disrupted cognitive functioning would manifest itself by impaired memory, difficulty in learning new material, and difficulty communicating with others. The quantification of these adverse effects requires neuropsychological assessments. Peripheral neuropathies would impair a person's sensory motor performance and would be a critical deficit in machine operators, cashiers, or anyone whose sense of touch is an important part of the job. In addition, these peripheral neuropathies may be related to impaired sexual functioning, with obvious implications for interpersonal relationships.

There are a wide variety of performance appraisal methods (including paper and pencil tests, direct observations, and simulation of work situations; Berk 1986), none of which are without limitations. Thus, a convergence in outcome of studies using different methods will be required for definitive conclusions. But what precisely would be expected to be the impact of cancer and its treatments on work performance? A representative set of outcomes would include the person performing his or her job slower, making more mistakes, having more accidents, having fewer sales, being less creative, setting unrealistic goals, not communicating well, not being cooperative, not coming to work on time, having an excessive number of sick days, or not having an average number of promotions over the course of his or her career. Also of interest is whether the employee's work performance reflects his or her response to co-workers, family, or personal psychological distress. How does the stigma of having cancer impact job dynamics and then the performance of the individual worker? These are just some of the issues that can be addressed by the performance appraisal process.

Worker-to-Job Fit

The congruence between job demands and the personal resources of the person (values, abilities, needs, motives, and goals), whether stated objectively or subjectively, is what is meant by worker-to-job fit (Locke 1976; Mortimer 1979). It has been hypothesized that the discrepancy between perceived job demands and perceived personal resources leads to work strain (French, et al. 1974, 1982). When the strain becomes excessive, it is expressed in such ways as job dissatisfaction, anxiety, depression or drug taking. Work strain also leads to body changes and, therefore, can impact the worker's health. These outcomes occur when the demands of the job exceed the capacities of the person leading to anxiety and low satisfaction, or when the person's capabilities may exceed the job's demand leading to boredom, depression, and low satisfaction.

The major limitation of studies of worker-to-job fit is that it has been difficult to develop a uniform and inclusive set of variables to describe the degree or extent of fit. Also, there is a tendency to assume that the extent of fit explains all (O'Brien 1986). Notwithstanding these limitations, there are distinct advantages in applying the worker-to-job fit research perspective to studies of the work history of the cancer patient. For example, the worker-to-job fit approach generates a difference measure (the difference between job demands and worker resources). This difference measure makes it possible to compare the heterogeneous population of workers and their jobs, ordinarily found in the population, along a common dimension.

One of the most consistent, but clinical, observations reported in the literature on the work history of the cancer patient is that major shifts in productive activities occur in individuals who are physically capable of continuing their pre-disease activities. These are clinical observations because there are no studies available in which the person's physical capacity was directly related to major changes in productive activities. One explanation of this observation is that the person with cancer feels that to continue to work, or engage in other forms of productive activity, somehow may actually worsen his or her health. A second advantage of the worker-to-job fit perspective is that it provides an appropriate theoretical framework to test this hypothesis. Thus, if fit is poor, then the worker will report job strain, and job strain may lead to poor health, as well as lower morale and productivity (O'Brien 1986). Could it be that the reason why a cancer patient retires early is because he or she feels his job may exacerbate illness? This hypothesis can be tested by correlating job strain to early retirement, or to a general lowering of productive activities. This study could be done with both objective and perceived measures of job strain, and any discrepancy between the two perspectives would be informative about the decision dynamics of the cancer patient.

Heilman's (1983) "lack-of-fit" model is an extension of the congruence hypothesis. Its application to the study of the discriminatory experience of the cancer patient was discussed in Chapter 1 (Barofsky, this volume). Fobair et al. (Chapter 6, this volume), used this method to examine their data. Its use prospectively to generate and test specific hypotheses has yet to be done. A particularly interesting research question is how much cancer-typing of jobs occurs. Are cancer patients excluded from certain types of jobs simply because of some misguided notion of the capabilities of the cancer patient? An example of this might be the systematic exclusion of laryngectomees from certain jobs because of concern of self-injury (e.g., because of dust).

Studies of Job Discrimination

Employment discrimination is a politically and economically unacceptable activity because it makes characteristics of the individual that are not relevant part of the work process. There are two sets of these characteristics: factors inherent or inseparable from the individual, such as the person's age, sex, and race, and then acquired factors, such as a person's ethnic or religious background, socioeconomic status, or disease status. A characteristic is acquired in that a person is not born in that state, and the state is at least modifiable, if not reversible. Acquired and inherent characteristics lead to analogous forms of discrimination because in both cases a person becomes a part of a subculture which includes a socialization process and distinctive group membership. Both groups also experience a bias in the assessment and evaluation processes.

Cancer is one type of chronic disease where it can be assumed that a proportion of the patients (i.e., patients with Hodgkin's disease, testicular patients, and certain stages of breast cancer) have a reasonable probability of living a normal life, either in terms of duration or functional status. There are, however, some cancer patients whose illness and treatment precludes work and these persons voluntarily withdrew from the work force. There are also persons whose incurable cancer has a natural history which permits the person to work, with little or no evidence of impairment, close to the time of death (e.g., colon or liver cancer). And there are, of course, patients whose disease is debilitating (e.g., the lung cancer patient), but who choose to work, even for the short periods available, to optimize their quality of life. There are also patients with clear physical limitations or disabilities who can be expected to have an extended survival.

Each of these classes of patients creates different contexts within which the issue of job discrimination has to be considered. Consider the issue of voluntary or involuntary departure from a job. It is generally considered that if a cancer patient is asked to leave a job, discrimination might be involved. Yet there are circumstances where asking the patient to leave may be legally and ethically defendable. At the same time there may be instances where an employer claims that accommodating a cancer patient's limitations may be excessive, when in fact it reflects a discriminatory intent.

In addition to different classes of cancer patients, there are also different theoretical approaches to job discrimination. In Chapter 1 (Barofsky, this volume) two basic approaches to job or employment discrimination were discussed: an economic and a social psychological perspective. Combining the classes of patients with the theoretical approaches generates a matrix each cell of which forms a natural research task.

Economic Models of Employment Discrimination

The free market approach to economics implies that it is acceptable to discriminate if it leads to greater productivity. If such discrimination is irrational, it will eventually become uneconomical (Becker 1957). Thus, if economic behavior is rational, discrimination will be limited to noneconomic forms (such as personal preferences).

One of the economic factors that leads to discrimination of employees is the capacity of the employee to adapt to changes in the person's work environment. This adaptability is referred to, in economic terms, as the "elasticity of the labor supply." One useful research question is to estimate how "elastic" the cancer patient is, as a subgroup of the labor supply. How adaptable are cancer patients, to what extent does this adaptability vary as a function of class of cancer patients (see above), and type of job? The answers to these questions could provide employers with objective information for formulating relatively rational personnel policies for the cancer patient.

An additional research question is to determine the extent to which employment discrimination can be accounted for in terms of intentional discrimination or cumulative causation (Barofsky [Chapter 1], this volume). In intentional discrimination there is a direct linkage between the attitudes and behaviors of the employer and instances of discrimination. This direct linkage suggests a linear causation model. In contrast, the cumulative causation model assumes an interaction between the employer and characteristics of the employee leading to more and more justification for discrimination. This model suggests the operation of a feedback process. The two models, however, would be expected to make different predictions and testing for these predictions would be useful not only for understanding the experience of the cancer patient but also for understanding employment discrimination, in general. The two models should also lead to different interventions.

Social Psychological Aspects of Employment Discrimination

There is an extensive literature dealing with sociological and psychological aspects of discrimination, a portion of which includes employment discrimination (e.g., Dovido & Gaertner 1986). There is very little literature dealing with these same issues for persons with various illnesses who become victims of job discrimination, although its application seems obvious and straightforward. Two examples will be given here to illustrate how the available social psychological literature can be applied to understand job discrimination of the cancer patient.

One of the more universal clinical observations is that patients seem to find someone who is worse off than they are among the patients they see and interact with. Whether the person has an amputation, face deformity, or whatever, there always is someone who is less fortunate than they are. What the person is doing when he does this is to distinguish him- or herself from others in such a way as to feel better in comparison to others. Social psychologists refer to this phenomenon as the "downward comparison principle" (Wills 1981). It is a principle that has received little formal study among cancer patients.

The theory of downward comparison states that persons can increase their subjective well-being through comparison with a less fortunate other. This process is evoked by negative affect. Thus, a downward comparison occurs when a decrease in subjective well-being occurs, or threat to self-esteem. Downward comparison can occur passively, when an opportunity arises, by active derogation, also called scapegoating, or by causing harm to a less fortunate person. Thus, clustered under the concept of downward comparison are a variety of interesting social psychological phenomena that can be tested in the context of job discrimination of the cancer patient. It is most useful that the same set of principles can be used to analyze the role of both the employer and employee in job discrimination. It could provide important insights into the self-limitation process that is hypothesized to occur among cancer patients (that is, self-limitation is actually a psychological method that cancer patients use to preserve their senses of self-esteem), as well as providing a psychological "explanation" for job discrimination by employers.

It has been amply documented by social scientists that stereotyping is a critical aspect of racial prejudice, discrimination, and intergroup relations. A stereotype is a generalization about a group that is applied to an individual. It would be expected to play a role in employment discrimination of the cancer patient. It may account for why good prognosis patients (e.g., Hodgkin's disease patients) report work-related problems and discrimination (Barofsky [Chapter 1], this volume).

Ashmore and Del Boca (1981) point out that there are three ways of conceiving of how stereotypes develop and are perpetuated. In one, stereotypes are viewed as a product of motivational processes; the product of intrapsychic conflict. In a second, it is seen as a product of social learning processes, and in a third, it is a cognitive category used by social perceivers in processing information about people. Each of these perspectives is associated with an elaborate literature (Dovido & Gaertner 1986).

There are a wide variety of research questions that can be asked about the role of stereotypes in employment discrimination of the cancer patient. First, would be to determine if stereotypes of the cancer patient exist, and how they developed. Second, it should be possible to design studies based on the three different theoretical models discussed. If, for example, a stereotype is a cognitive categorization, then it should be possible to determine the stimuli that are used to classify people into different categories.

Elements of an Interventions Program

In Chapter 1 (Barofsky, this volume) it was made clear that almost from the time of McKenna's (1973) report describing the adverse work and insurance history of the cancer patient, plans were being made to design and implement interventions. It was assumed that definitions of and interventions designed for correcting racial and ethnic discrimination could be applied to the problem of job discrimination of the cancer patient. The results of the National Cancer Institute–sponsored Work-able Project demonstrated that this assumption was incorrect (see Chapter 1).

In its stead an admixture of methods and approaches has evolved that applies definitions of employment discrimination of the disabled (e.g., the

Rehabilitation Act of 1973, and state and local laws) to the cancer patient. This approach doesn't cover the most blatant examples of job discrimination which involve persons with cancer with no disability. As a result, congressional initiatives have appeared to provide a more comprehensive legal basis for barring employment discrimination in the cancer patient.

Most instances of job discrimination are identified by complaints lodged by individual cancer patients. These types of complaints, however, are quite rare. For example, Brighaim (1979) found that during the period from 1974 to 1978 only 1.3 percent of complaints under the Rehabilitation Act of 1973 were by cancer patients. In addition, Barofsky (1982), reported that only two court cases involved cancer patients prior to 1982, although since then there has been a substantial increase in the number of cancer-related litigations.

These data raise questions regarding whether or not job and insurance discrimination of the cancer patient is an occasional event that can be dealt with after it has been identified, or if it occurs sufficiently often to justify some national, or even local, interventions that are targeted at employers (as was planned in the National Cancer Institute's Work-able Project). Neither option can be selected, however, in the absence of adequate data on the incidence and prevalence of employment discrimination of the cancer patient. But even if the number of individuals affected justified the cost of an intervention much has to be learned about how to design and implement the intervention, and what statistical approaches can be used to assess the outcome of the intervention.

The Epidemiology of Work Adjustment

Most studies of the work history of the cancer patient consist of convience samples which provide retrospective self-reports of work experiences. They clearly cannot be used to provide population-based estimates of work-related problems.

The study which comes closest to providing these type of data was reported by Houts, et al. (Chapter 5, this volume but also Houts, et al. 1986). Houts, et al., interviewed 629 newly diagnosed cancer patients obtained from a state tumor registry to determine their unmet needs. He then used these data to generate population-based (the population of the state of Pennsylvania) estimates of the number of persons with particular unmet needs. He estimated that approximately 56,000 persons in the state will develop cancer in one year. Of these 56,000 persons with cancer only 7 percent (or 4000 persons) report work-related problems, but 20 percent of the persons who worked following their diagnosis, report work-related problems. These data, of course, do not include persons who have had cancer (prevalence data), nor is it appropriate to classify a work-related problem as being the same as having a discriminatory experience.

Determining the epidemiology of work adjustment generates a number of study problems. For example, it will be necessary to rapidly identify patients who are diagnosed with cancer and were working prior to disease onset, if a representative sample is to be followed prospectively. Most tumor registries identify cases within months of diagnosis so that a delay may be inherent to using the registries as a case identification source.

In addition, if the method used by Houts, et al. is used to identify persons with work problems it would be inappropriate to assume that they were having a discriminatory experience. One of the purposes of this book, however, was to alert investigators to the fact that having a problem at work because of cancer may still justify an intervention, although the intervention may not include efforts at legal redress. Thus, a study of this sort can be justified on the basis of estimating the rate work-related problems occur in the presence of cancer, some of which may be discriminatory in nature. By focusing the research on work-related problems, the investigators may simplify their definitional task since they can restrict the definition of job discrimination to those work-related problems which require litigation for resolution, or match some state or federal definition of discrimination.

Design Issues

If an investigator accepts the view that job discrimination is at one extreme of what is a continuum of work-related problems, then a study can be performed which would determine the impact of cancer on the frequency of work-related problems. Work-related problems include an excessive number of sick days, difficulties with co-workers, reduced productivity, physical limitations, and so on. The hypothesis to be tested is that having cancer results in an increase in the frequency of work-related problems. To an extent, the research of Houts, et al. (1986), has already confirmed this hypothesis, although without the level of specificity required to pinpoint the exact nature of the impact of cancer on work history. The same arguments can be made for studies of other forms of productive activities.

What an intervention program will look like cannot be specified at this time. It is not even clear that a national or local campaign needs to be mounted. Instead, a system may be developed which permits interventions for individual cases. Hays (1986) and his colleagues have developed such a program. They are in the process of evaluating a system that uses volunteers who are critically involved in personnel matters (personnel directors, hiring agents, employers) or insurance matters (medical directors, underwriters, actuaries) to intervene in individual cases. Their approach is simple and direct, but will be useful only if the frequency of work-related problems is small enough for a volunteer board to manage. If not, then other types of interventions may be required.

What would be an appropriate control group for an intervention study? Houts, et al. and Teta (Chapters 5 & 3, this volume) used siblings of the patients as controls. Most other studies of the work history of the cancer patient do not include a control group. The control groups that can be used include the patient's siblings, co-workers, persons with the same job but not working for the same employer, workers in general, workers with different chronic diseases, and members of the general population. Each control group would provide a different answer to the question of whether cancer increased the frequency of work-related problems. The patient's sibling is the control of choice, since he or she would likely match the patient in terms of socioeconomic status, occupation, or exposure to a "cancer" environment. Exposure to a cancer environment, however, may compromise the sibling's work experience so that it would also be necessary to include a control group of, say, co-workers whose work history would be totally free of such effects. A study involving both types of control groups has not been reported to date.

Statistical Issues

The Work-able Project made it clear that an actuarial definition of job discrimination of the cancer patient was not feasible. It is not possible to state, as one can for race, sex, or age, that the difference in the percent of the general population with cancer who are working, and that of cancer patients working at work site "A" is evidence of employment discrimination. Part of the reason this is so is because it is difficult to estimate the prevalence of cancer in the general population. Primarily, because it has not been technically possible to declare a person cured of cancer and no longer countable. In addition, the small number of persons who have work-related problems increases the chances of errors in any estimate of work-related problems.

An innovative measurement approach would apply stochastic modeling (Diekman & Mitter 1984) to work history data. The advantage of a stochastic approach is that work history would be conceptualized in dynamic as opposed to static terms. In addition, outcomes would be stated in probabilistic not deterministic terms. Stochastic modeling, for example, would provide estimates of the transition probabilities associated with a cancer patient shifting between specific jobs, between a job and no job, between a job and other forms of productive activities. By combining standard regression analyses (Allison 1984) with stochastic modeling, it will also be possible to identify the factors that are associated with state changes (e.g., having a job and then shifting to another form of productive activity).

A third advantage of stochastic modeling is that it presents data in terms of time a person is in a particular state, or the frequency with which events occur. This avoids many of the arbitrary psychological scales and dimensions, and can be considered a step in the direction of formulating general behavioral laws (Rapoport 1984).

SUMMARY

Employment discrimination has been conceptualized in this book in at least two ways: as a strong and a weak model. In the weak model job discrimination was considered present if cancer became part of the work history of an individual. Thus, if a person's career or insurance premiums were adversely affected because the person had cancer, and this did not occur for persons who did not have cancer, then this was considered discriminatory. In the strong model, job discrimination was considered present only if it was legally demonstrated or met some legal definition of discrimination, without having to be adjudicated. No decision could be made on which definition of job discrimination to use because of the lack of consensus in the literature on whether the discriminatory experiences the cancer patients report are psychological (something the person feels) or institutional/organizational in nature. It was also made clear that the definition of employment discrimination would vary as a function of level of analysis: economic or social/psychological.

The Declaration of Independence states that "all men are created equal." While a political statement, this statement also has economic implications (Edwin 1986)—the economic implications being that one of the goals of this society is that every individual be given the opportunity to achieve economic security, independent of his or her work-ableness. Job discrimination prevents this from happening, whether it is a cancer patient or a minority group member who is the victim. In either case, it contradicts the objectives of this society so that it should become an object of remediation.

This chapter was designed to whet the appetite of investigators. It was not meant to be definitive or even comprehensive; many topics could have been included as proposed research which were not, and their absence should be taken as a statement of irrelevance, rather selective perception.

REFERENCES

Allison, P. D. Event history analysis: Regression for longitudinal event data. Beverly Hills, CA: Sage, 1984.

Ashmore, R. D., & Del Boca, F. K. Conceptual approaches to stereotypes and stereotyping. In D. L. Hamilton (Ed.), Cognitive processes in stereotyping and intergroup behavior. Hillsdale, N.J.: Erlbaum, 1981, pp. 1–35.

Barofsky, I. Job discrimination: A measure of the social death of the cancer patient. Proceedings of the western states conference on cancer rehabilitation.. Palo Alto, CA: Bull, 1982.

Becker, G. S. The economics of discrimination. Chicago: University of Chicago, 1957.

Bergermaier, R., Borg, I., & Champoux, J. E. Structural relationships among facets of work, nonwork and general well-being. Work and Occupation, 1984, 11, 163–181.

Berk, R. A. *Performance assessment: Methods and applications.* Baltimore, MD: Johns Hopkins, 1986.

Bray, D. W., & Howard, A. The AT&T longitudinal study of managers. In K. W. Schaie (Ed.), *Longitudinal studies of adult psychological development.* New York: Guilford, 1983.

Brighaim, D. Personal communication, 1979.

Brouwers, P., Riccardi, R., Fedio, P., & Poplack, D. G. Long term neuropsychological sequelae of childhood cancer leukemia: Correlation with CT brain scan abnormalities. *Journal of Pediatrics,* 1985, *106,* 723–730.

Cancer Statistics. *CA—A Cancer Journal for Clinicians.* 1988, *38,* 5–22.

Diekmann, A., & Mitter, P. *Stochastic modeling of social processes.* Orlando, FL: Academic, 1984.

Dovido, J. F., & Gaertner, S. L. *Prejudice, discrimination and racism.* Orlando, FL: Academic, 1986.

Edwin, D. Personal communication, 1987.

Feldman, F. L. *Work and cancer health histories: A study of the experiences of recovered blue-collar workers.* Oakland: California Division, American Cancer Society, 1978.

Feldman, J. J. *Work ability of the aged under conditions of improved mortality.* Statement before the National Commission on Social Security Reform. June 1982.

Freedman, M. The search for shelters. In K. Thompson (Ed.), *Work, employment and unemployment.* Milton Keynes: The Open University Press, 1984, pp. 55–66.

French, J. R. P., Caplan, R. D., & Harrison, R. V. *The mechanisms of job stress and strain.* Chichester: Wiley, 1982.

French, J. R. P., Rogers, W., & Cobb, S. A model of person-environment fit. In G. V. Coelho, D. A. Hamburgh, & J. E. Adams (Eds.), *Coping and adaptation.* New York: Basic Books, 1974.

Hayes, J., & Nutman, P. *Understanding the unemployed: The psychological effects of unemployment.* London: Tavistock, 1981.

Hays, D. M. *Aiding childhood cancer patients confront adult issues.* Grant Application to the National Cancer Institute, March 1986.

Heilman, M. E. Sex bias in work settings: The lack of fit model. *Research and Organizational Behavior,* 1983, *5,* 269–298.

Hogan, J., & Quigley, A. M. Physical standards for employment and the courts. *American Psychologist,* 1986, *41,* 1193–1227.

Houts, P., Yasko, J., Kahn, S. B., Schelzel, G., & Marconi, K. Unmet psychological, social and economic needs of persons with cancer in Pennsylvania. *Cancer,* 1986, *58,* 2355–2361.

Koral, A. M. Practical application of the Uniform Guidelines: What to do 'till the agency comes. *Employee Relations Law Journal,* 1980, *5,* 473–492.

Littler, C. R. *The development of the labour process in capitalist societies: A comparative analysis of work organization in Britain, the U.S.A. and Japan.* London: Heinemann, 1982.

Locke, E. A. The nature and causes of job satisfaction. In M. D. Dunnette (Ed.), *Handbook of industrial and organizational psychology.* Chicago: Rand McNally, 1976.

Mages, N. L. & Mendelsohn, G. A. Effects of cancer on patients' lives: A personological approach. In G. C. Stone, F. Cohen, & N. E. Adler (Eds.), *Health Psychology*. San Francisco: Jossey-Bass, 1979.

McKenna, R. J. *Analysis of case histories: Re-employment problems of the recovered cancer patient. A report by the Ad Hoc Subcommittee on Employability Problems of the Recovered Cancer Patient*. San Francisco: American Cancer Society, Inc., California Division, 1973.

Medical Standards Project. *A new approach: The individual assessment hiring procedure, a handbook for employing disabled persons*. San Francisco: Unpublished, 1983.

Mellette, S. J., & Franco, P. C. Psychosocial barriers to employment of the cancer survivor. *Journal of Psychosocial Oncology*, 1987, 5, 97–115.

Mortimer, J. T. *Changing attitudes toward work*. Scarsdale, NY: Work in America Institute, 1979.

O'Brien, G. E. *Psychology of work and unemployment*. New York: Wiley, 1986.

O'Brien, G. E., Dowling, P., & Kabanoff, B. *Work, health, and leisure*. National Institute of Labour Studies, Working Paper 28, Adelaide, The Flinders University of South Australia, 1978.

Parkes, C. M. Psychosocial transitions: A field of study. *Social Science and Medicine*, 1971, 5, 101–115.

Parkes, C. M. The emotional impact of cancer on patients and families. *Journal of Laryngology and Otology*, 1975, 89, 1271–1279.

Phillips, S. L., Pizzo P., & Gerber, L. Work status of childhood cancer survivors. Presented at the Tenth Annual Mental Health Conference, M. D. Anderson Hospital and Tumor Institute. April 1985.

Rapoport, A. New aspects of stochastic model building in the social sciences. In A. Diekmann & P. Mitter (Eds.), *Stochastic modeling of social processes*. Orlando, FL: Academic, 1984.

Salaman, G. *Working*. London: Tavistock, 1986.

Scott, J. B. Practical aspects of fair employment litigation. *Public Personnel Management*, 1977, 6, 398–406.

Wills, T. A. Downward comparison principles in social psychology. *Psychological Bulletin*, 1981, 90, 245–271.

Zubin, J., & Spring, B. Vulnerability—A new view of schizophrenia. *Journal of Abnormal Psychology*, 1977, 86, 103–126.

9

Maximizing the Productive Activities of the Cancer Patient: Policy Issues

Robert J. McKenna and Nicholas J. Toghia

Cancer is our most common chronic illness and more than 5 million Americans are now alive after the diagnosis of cancer. Each year, another 1 million Americans will be newly diagnosed with cancer. The overall cure rate of cancer is now 51 percent and is improving each year. Dr. DeVita, the former director of the National Cancer Institute, projects that the cure rate will be 75 percent by the year 2000 (DeVita 1986). This improvement is dependent on the successful prevention of cancer due to known carcinogens, the application of new knowledge in the detection and screening for cancer at an early stage, and the continuing improvement in treatment of cancer by surgery, radiotherapy, and/or chemotherapy with hopes that immunotherapy will soon be added to this list.

Notwithstanding these strides, the lay public and employers view the diagnosis of cancer with great pessimism, if not with the expectation of a fatal outcome. The prior statistics would certainly imply a favorable prognosis for the majority and one that is constantly improving and will continue to improve. It should be emphasized that those individuals who are not completely cured of their cancer are frequently able to survive for many years in a state of relatively good health and able to work and lead a good quality life. Although nearly half of all cancer occurs in Americans who are either retired or in school, most of the remainder are employed at the time of the cancer diagnosis and, after treatment, over 80 percent of these individuals are able to return to productive work activity.

It should be emphasized that cancer is not one disease, but a group of diseases affecting many different organ sites in the body with the ability to produce a range of alteration in life-style from none to total disability. The diversity is, in part, defined by the stage of cancer—from early to regional to far advanced when first diagnosed—and also by the organ site involved. For example, breast cancer, frequently diagnosed at a very early stage, may be treated conservatively and will rarely create a problem with disability unless extensive metastases occur. At the other extreme, pancreas cancer is rarely cured, early diagnosis is nearly nonexistent and the progression of symptoms is such that disability occurs early, is rapidly progressive, and rarely allows one the ability to return to work or to enjoy a good quality of life. A type of an in-between site might be colon cancer, where approximately half are diagnosed at an early stage and treatment is usually quite successful. Surgical removal allows the patient to return to work in a period of six to eight weeks with no significant or noticeable disability and with a fairly good prognosis for the long term. Imagine if you will, a hundred different cancer types and sites of varying stages and diverse prognoses, and it follows that each patient needs not only individualized treatment but also varying degrees of rehabilitation to return to a near normal life-style including work activity.

This book is devoted to a comprehensive discussion of the broad implications of cancer as an illness and its impact on work. The basic issues and salutary effects of work are described by Barofsky (Chapter 1, this volume). Through the years the ethos of work has changed; in our industrialized society it became specialized, goal oriented, and increasingly more competitive. In this atmosphere, unfortunately, a history of a cancer illness does nothing to improve one's potential for gainful employment and can interfere with work performance if the duration of medical care is prolonged or if treatment complications result. Frequently, it can have a major impact on work performance should a recurrence of cancer or metastases occur. Job performance is the litmus test of employee work effort, and it may be affected when the employee loses interest in living or in his job and is also impacted by decreased stamina due to illness.

With this preamble in mind, we strongly believe that the time has come for employers, large and small, public and private, to deal with the role of the rehabilitated cancer patient in the work force (Table 9.1). To achieve this objective will require a massive attitude adjustment at the highest levels of corporate management in America. Further, we must embrace maximizing the productive activities of the cancer patient as a matter of public policy for the nation. At the minimum, based on its own observation and analysis of its work force, any sizable business must assess the degree to which it needs to be involved in an appropriate program, given the fact that different legal standards are applicable to public and private employment practices. The issue is the subject of intense current debate, legislative efforts, and increasing litigation. Eventually, we hope, distinctions between public and private employers will be eliminated and all sectors will implement similar and harmonious treatment of the cancer patient in the work force.

To avoid a patchwork quilt approach to this problem, a rational and systematic framework will be necessary. We suggest that a workable approach for the employer would be to:

1. Adopt a company policy against discrimination in the hiring, training, promotion, and compensation of the work-able cancer patient;

2. Familiarize management with the requirements of federal and state statutes, as well as court cases, with the assistance of in-house counsel or outside attorneys;

3. Articulate and design a sensible program that fits the company's needs, using input from a variety of sources including human resources staff, departmental supervisors, company medical personnel, health care providers, the National Cancer Institute, and the American Cancer Society;

4. Monitor on a systematic basis the company's experience with the program to gather reliable statistics to dispel the misconceptions that the rehabilitated cancer patient is less productive, more expensive, and, therefore, a less valuable member of the work force than the rest of the employees;

5. Evaluate the program at periodic intervals to determine if modifications or improvements should be implemented;

6. Acknowledge and publicize the success of the program to boost employee morale and to improve the work atmosphere within the organization; and

7. Broaden the impact of the program by encouraging participation of other employers in like programs at their companies via contacts through trade associations, chambers of commerce, local press, and the media.

BROAD PARAMETERS OF THE PROBLEM

Feldman (Chapter 2, this volume) has stated that "to work is to survive, to be independent and to be self-sufficient; to earn is a measure of personal adequacy and worth." She raises complex issues of work ability and describes this as the fit between the individual's work skills and available and accessible work opportunities, the constellation of the worker's personal qualities, and their compatibility with conditions and persons in the workplace, and a host of other factors. The assessment of the work ability of the individual with a cancer history is compounded by social and emotional attitudes rooted in antiquity that may threaten the recovered person's ability to be in the work force and, indeed, his or her very quality of life.

The economic burden of cancer impacts upon the employer, the employee, his family, and society in general. This nation's total economic burden of cancer is staggering and is estimated to amount to $65.2 billion (Rice, et al. 1987) in 1985; 28 percent or $18.1 billion of these total figures are due to direct costs of medical care including hospital and nursing home

Table 9.1
Checklist for Employers Willing to Implement Nondiscriminatory
Programs to Hire Workers with a History of Cancer Illness

1. Gather relevant data on attendance, productivity, health care usage, accidents and workers compensation claims for both employers affected by cancer as well as those unaffected by the illness and compare the statistics to verify if there are substantial differences.

2. Confront potential dilemmas and decide in advance how you will handle them.

3. Question if it is in the company's long-term business interest to deny employment to, or terminate,all individuals when they are diagnosed with a cancer problem even when they are superior performers.

4. Question if it is in the firm's long range economic interest to deny hiring or rehiring, training or promotion to cancer patients despite the fact they are work able and are otherwise qualified.

5. Avoid differentiation between high and low level employees when administering the program--there should be equal treatment for all jobs, from president to janitor.

6. Disseminate company policies in writing to employees and state company philosophy in as many ways as possible: employment application, employee handbook, insurance information, bulletin board notices, company newsletters, etc.

Table 9.1 Continued

7. Train supervisors to deal effectively with employees who may be experiencing problems of discrimination or abuse from co-workers because their cancer condition is a matter of common knowledge at the work place.

8. Develop reasonable performance standards that may include flexible work hours, shortened work days, assistance with commuting from home to work, car pooling, etc.

9. Apply company policies consistently and reasonably and reassure employees that if their job performance is satisfactory, job security will not be jeopardized solely because of their medical condition.

10. If the company is unionized, involve the union to defuse and mitigate against potential labor trouble due to improper or unjustified termination, reassignment, demotion, denial or reduction of benefits.

11. Become aware of legal ramifications and potential statutory and common law liability: wrongful discharge; breach of employment contract; implied covenant of good faith and fair dealing, infliction of emotional distress; defamation.

Source: Compiled by the authors.

care, services of physicians and other health professionals, and drugs. More than 60 percent of the total cost of cancer is due to mortality costs—the value of losses due to premature deaths from cancer. Morbidity costs, which include the value of lost productivity due to illness and disability for patients suffering from cancer, amounted to $7.1 billion or 11 percent of the total cancer costs in the United States in 1985. Cancer, the second leading cause of death in the United States, took 457,600 lives in 1985. The average cost per cancer death amounted to $87,000. More than a third (157,400 persons) who died from this disease were under the age of 65—their most productive years—and costs per death in this group amounted to $114,600 per capita.

Although about 90 percent of Americans are covered by some form of health insurance, cancer may often be a catastrophic illness with devastatingly adverse financial consequences for individuals and their families. Congress is presently addressing this issue, where cost of medical care has produced an unreasonable burden for the patient with cancer. It is obvious that those persons without health care coverage who develop cancer are often faced with a peculiarly difficult economic crisis. Their ability to obtain and pay for adequate treatment and care is severely limited. Of those who are insured, most individuals are covered by group health insurance rather than individual insurance and this is obtained normally through their employment, paid for in part or in whole by the employer. Health care coverage is clearly the most important fringe benefit derived from employment. The opportunity to continue health care coverage on an individual basis is usually available but often may not be recognized or arranged for by the employee until it is too late. Once lost, getting new coverage with a preexisting condition such as a history of cancer is extremely difficult. Hence, being able to work has not only the economic benefits of providing an adequate living for the worker and his family, but has the hidden advantage of offering group health insurance for coverage of future health impairments. If the patient does not return to work after cancer treatment, industry will lose a much needed worker, government loses taxes, and potentially an additional family is placed on the welfare rolls. The dilemma of rehabilitation of a cancer patient is a joint responsibility of all society.

Most patients who have been treated for cancer want to return to work, are able to return to work, and should be encouraged to do so. Problems facing the cancer patient when he or she returns to work may include accommodating any change in functional ability, the attitude of the employer, and the often subtle actions of co-workers. Considerable data on employment is presented in this book in chapters by Feldman; Teta; Holmes, et al.; Fobiar, et al.; Houts, et al.; and Ganz, et al. Other references are listed in individual chapters as well. Unless one were able to monitor the work history of all individuals diagnosed with cancer for a number of years after diagnoses are made and treatment given, one can only postulate about the true incidence of problems associated with employment. It is clear from the studies to date that a problem does exist, that it is probably understated, that it is more common for the blue-collar worker than for the white-collar worker, and that it is more common among those earning a low salary.

SALUTARY EFFECTS OF WORK UPON THE CANCER PATIENT

It has always been our opinion that everyone with a cancer diagnosis should be able to return to work if work-able and that, if necessary, some accommodation be made for those who need modification of their job description. The issue of return to work is rarely of paramount importance when the cancer diagnosis is made. At that time the individual often asks: Why did cancer happen to me? Will I survive? What is the optimum treatment for my stage of cancer? Will I have complications or disability from the planned treatment? And often, Can I afford care? It is clearly the responsibility of the treating physician and the cancer rehabilitation team to discuss with the patient the date when work may be resumed and, if disability exists, how this may be overcome in order to be able successfully to return to employment. The individual needs to be encouraged to set his or her goal regarding return to work and not milk the system for unnecessary sick leave, disability benefits, and unemployment compensation. The incentive is high when the job is satisfying, and the reverse is true when compensation is low and the job is boring. We believe it is an error to seek early retirement or prolonged disability in many cases where the oncology nurse or the social worker may think that the prognosis may be less favorable. The premise for this opinion is that one cannot always prognosticate cancer outcome and many individuals with what appears to be a very poor prognosis live for many years with a good quality of life. It is often very difficult to return to employment once one has elected to quit the work force. Job counseling should be a part of the cancer rehabilitation effort. Some individuals, such as a laryngectomee, need vocational rehabilitation and this should be actively pursued to ensure adequate speech for communication. The amputee needs to minimize the delay in fitting a prosthesis, learning its use, and not procrastinate, as was commonplace years ago when the prevailing attitude was wait and see whether one survives cancer before a prosthesis is fitted.

On return to work, it might be ideal if part-time employment could be arranged for those with fatigue or some disability, but this often is not the case in our modern industrial society. Accommodation may be more feasible in small firms and is more likely for the white-collar than the blue-collar worker. The most socialist of countries will not encourage (and even discourage) return to work for long periods or forever.

Adjuvant therapy for patients with cancer is often applied in the form of radiation therapy or chemotherapy and may be given over a period of months or up to a year. This most often is given on an outpatient basis in the office or clinic and often requires only a few hours per week away from work. The employer needs to understand the need for this treatment and the inconvenience that may result, but should understand the psychological benefits accrued by returning to work, if possible, during such treatment, both for economic and psychosocial reasons. The system breaks down when there is a lack of communications or understanding between the employee and the employer and it is at this point that the attending physician needs to provide responsible medical input to assist the employer in understanding the problem and assist the employee in returning to work. In periods of high unemployment one could suggest replacing the worker but this requires training, the loss of an experienced employee, and often the imposition of a major economic burden on the employee and his family. Loyalty of the employee as well as the employer is sometime lost during any economic crunch. We think it is unconscionable to consider dismissing the employee because of a history of cancer but such is the case all too frequently in our modern world. The loss of health insurance coverage due to the whims of the employer seems unfair and is usually prevented by law.

A variety of other discriminatory practices may occur and are well spelled out by Feldman in Chapter 2. In a study by Mor (1986), a sample of 297 lung, breast, and colorectal cancer patients under age 65 were studied, 75 percent of whom were employed at the time of cancer diagnosis and remained employed six months later. Most of those who were no longer able to work were either lung cancer patients or patients with metastases. Most (72%) remained employed six months post-diagnosis suggesting that the functional status was the major factor in determining whether patients remained employed. A surprising fact was that 17 percent of those who were still employed had a significant change in their health insurance coverage due to decreased benefits.

A practical measure which can optimize the quality of life of the cancer patient is public education to erase archaic ideas that equate stigma, immorality, and contagion with cancer. This information approach has rarely been done in the work setting for the employer and is especially appropriate for the gatekeeper: medical director, personnel office, and anyone who makes decisions about permitting a patient to return to work after an illness. Similar education is appropriate for those in the workplace with whom the returning patient comes in contact so that there will not be any of the subtle negative behavior that is rarely openly stated but not infrequently pervades the workplace. The patient returning to work is faced with a dilemma as to whether he or she should or should not speak of the recent illness to both employer and fellow employees. The rumor mill can spread mistruths like wildfire and is often exaggerated after repeated conversations among the work force. Hostile situations may be encountered by the employee on a return to the labor force. The help of a professional counselor or a support network will prepare the employee to answer either explicit or implicit questions about cancer. In this way, depression may often be avoided when an individual is work-able and encounters such situations in the work force. Work remains a measure of adequacy and a way to meet obligations— financial, social, and psychological. The individual may have little control of the outcome of cancer treatment but work, when it is satisfying, clearly represents a self-fulfillment that is needed by most individuals. The Feldman study (Chapter 2) showed that over 50 percent of the white-collar workers, 84 percent of the blue-collar workers, and about 25 percent of the students had problems either in the workplace or in school. This has commonly been called a form of discrimination. Perhaps it would be better to avoid this word since it has negative implications. A positive approach is the solution to this dilemma. Should these problems be impossible to resolve through education, statutory protection of the law exists in most states for some workers and is currently under consideration by Congress. This would offer a legal remedy to persons discriminated against in the workplace because of a cancer history. It is our opinion that the ultimate most satisfying solution is the education of both employer and employee.

VOCATIONAL REHABILITATION

Public rehabilitative agencies have long been available for a wide range of services for individuals with illnesses, disabilities, and late effects of trauma. Surprisingly, few state agencies, however, carry much of a cancer caseload. Sheppard (1986) of the Michigan Rehabilitation Services reports that only 6 percent of their caseload is for patients with cancer; 93 percent of these are self-referred. The largest number of these patients are laryngectomees who need speech therapy to allow them to communicate and to compete in this vocal world. Most rehabilitation agencies are frustrated because of the low referral rate of cancer patients in spite of the high success rate of employment of such individuals. Some have suggested the use of the term *cancer rehabilitation* to increase public exposure and awareness, but the referral of patients to such agencies may create anxiety among employers and misunderstanding on the part of the oncologic physicians. Some vocational rehabilitation agencies have so little exposure to the cancer patient that their experience remains quite limited. The targeted objective is to achieve a good quality of life; the performance of functions of independent living; and the ability to return to work with or without job accommodations that might require a change in the work environment, a change in the flow of work, or a change in job duties. The ultimate solution may be sharing of resources among public rehabilitation agencies, hospital facilities, and voluntary health organizations such as the American Cancer Society in a team approach to maximize and broaden success through such progress.

WORK SITE COUNSELING

Today in the work force, there is a significant interest in health promotion and illness prevention with the belief in the corporate world that this will provide healthier employees and less absenteeism. We discussed earlier how there were some prejudicial attitudes founded on fear, anxiety, and ignorance facing both survivors and their employers. A pilot project was undertaken by Cancer Care, Inc. in New York City to undertake work site counseling and consultation to identify and assist employers and employees in resolving a wide range of cancer-related issues that can occur in the workplace (Leeds 1986). Although this program has had limited application in the country to date, the preliminary assessment of this demonstration project is that it has been beneficial. Some of their educational and training seminars have been conducted for unions and other groups in the corporate world to solve or prevent occurrences in the workplace that might be real and functional and others that could be based only on myth.

AMERICAN CANCER SOCIETY ROLE IN EMPLOYABILITY

For more than 25 years concerns with employment of the cancer patient has been an agenda item of the American Cancer Society (ACS). The problems of employability have been discussed through a variety of workshops and seminars sponsored by the ACS. Many issues in employability have not always been made public by the employee and considerable public education has been necessary to make the cancer patient aware of his or her rights in the workplace. Publications about performance in the workplace have demonstrated that patients with a cancer health history can do their fair share of work, with lower turnover and absenteeism rates than other employees. In some studies, their productivity is better than that of the average employee. There is much publicity about the many people who are now living with cancer and who can enjoy full and productive years if cured and even if not cured.

In November 1983, the ACS issued a policy statement stating, "although most people treated for cancer will be functionally unchanged, an individual with a history of cancer may need to be considered disabled or handicapped in order to seek protection under the law in the area of employment or insurance discrimination." Disability, when applied to the cancer patient, is a condition resulting in a loss or a decrease in ability to function effectively in one or more specific areas as a result of an impairment due to cancer or its treatment. The disability may be real or may be perceived as a disability by the individual. If the individual is unable to function in a required environment, he may further be considered handicapped as a result of his disability. In contrast to individuals disabled or handicapped by injury or birth defects, the cancer patient may have a "dynamic" disability. The degree of disability in such patients will be affected by exacerbation or remission of the cancer and/or its treatment, and include the probability of returning to near normal function.

Protection under the law is covered by Sections 503 and 504 of the Rehabilitation Act of 1973. Section 503 applies to most employers doing contract business with the federal government. Employers must hire handicapped persons and they cannot discriminate when hiring, promoting, transferring, recruiting, laying off, terminating, paying or selecting them for training. About half of all the nation's businesses are covered. The limitations of this Act are that it clearly does not cover all employees and it often requires a prolonged legal battle to resolve an issue which should have never happened. Section 504 of the Rehabilitation Act calls for nondiscrimination in every type of institution that receives federal funds; examples are schools, colleges, or hospitals.

Under the law, employment criteria must be job-related and measurable, not based on disability. Prospective employees cannot be asked to have a physical or medical examination before a job is offered. A physical or health questionnaire may be required after a job is offered only if it is also required for all other applicants. At times a pre-employment tryout or job tryout may be required to determine if the person can do job-related tasks.

The problem that occurs frequently with the application of this statute is that many patients who have had cancer do not consider themselves disabled but they need to be so designated to seek protection under this statute. Many patients who have had cancer do not consider themselves handicapped even though they may have lost an extremity, had a laryngectomy or even had a colostomy.

In 1986 Congress passed a unanimous resolution in both Houses stating that employment discrimination against cancer survivors was not to be condoned. While this resolution is a nonbinding statement of intent by Congress and not a formal statute, its passage signifies an important development in outlawing employment injustice.

At present, the ACS is funding a cancer control grant to the Legal Aid Society of San Francisco for the purpose of providing information and training to ACS staff and volunteers on the illegal treatment of cancer survivors in the workplace. Protection under the law is extremely spotty and Delaware has no law for legal protection for the patient with cancer who experiences employment discrimination. In Alabama and Idaho only public employees are covered. In some states, the law is so vague that cancer is not mentioned and only the words "medical condition" are included. The state of Washington covers most employers with eight or more employees, and in California and Oregon the law covers most employers with five or more employees. We are in a period of transition of the law which we believe will be more crystallized in the coming years. The most difficult areas arise where the government is the employer; the armed forces has almost never accepted a new recruit with a past history of cancer even when no disability or evidence of disease is present. This has changed somewhat quite recently. The hiring at the city, county, state, and federal levels of a person with a cancer health history is more liberal now than it was 20 years ago but still has numerous restrictions and uneven application of fairness.

Thus, *the employment problem of the cancer patient is really a civil rights issue* with all the emotion usually generated by such matters. Education is clearly the solution to prevent the occurrence of discrimination in employment but this will take time. The uneven application of Sections 503 and 504 of the Rehabilitation Act needs to be clarified and expanded. This will require continued lobbying for new legislation. It may require 100 or 10,000 more employees so affected to come forth with their stories. We believe this is a cause that should be in the forefront of social legislation and one should continue to overcome this form of discrimination much of which is based on ignorance and misconception.

SEEKING NEW EMPLOYMENT AFTER CANCER

Getting a new job represents quite a different problem from keeping the old job. The number of job rejections attributed to cancer has been significant. Feldman reported 22 percent of the white collar workers, 45 percent of the blue collar workers and 45 percent of the youth experienced job rejections. These statistics vary widely in numerous other studies. Job rejection is not a factor if the cancer health history is not reported. It is possible that the disease may be used as a scapegoat for employment rejection. In some situations employers are unwilling to take a chance for fear the cancer may recur. Since so many factors are involved in the selection for employment, it is very difficult to appraise the true rate of rejection. Very few employers will now admit that they would use cancer as a basis for rejection though this was commonplace 25 years ago. Failure to get new employment means that the individual is locked into his present job and is often not able to advance in salary or job responsibility and is often limited in mobility to other areas to seek employment. The transferability of fringe benefits such as health insurance would go a long way to make it more possible for employees to be mobile and switch positions. The current insurance market with changing health delivery systems becoming more competitive makes the future somewhat unpredictable. We would hesitate to predict that employment problems of the individual with a cancer health history may be a long way from being totally solved and may be with us for many decades to come.

HEALTH INSURANCE COVERAGE

Over eight hundred insurance companies provide medical expense insurance and disability income insurance to well over 160 million people in the United States. Eighty-five percent of those so insured are working on the date the policy becomes effective and are covered through group plans without regard to health status. Fifteen percent have individual health insurance policies based on health criteria provided by carriers. In 1983, approximately 179 million had surgical coverage, 173 million had physician coverage, 162 million had major medical coverage, 64 million had short-term disability and 23 million had long-term disability insurance. Approximately 18.6 percent were uninsured or underinsured. This figure seems to be rising with changes in employment using more part-time workers often without insurance benefits.

The best way to protect insurance coverage is to try to return to work and not to take early retirement or disability. If employment is terminated due to disability, group insurance can be continued on an individual basis with an increased premium providing such is converted during the stated period, often 30 days. On an individual basis, the premium will be increased and often there will be a waiting period before being effective.

New coverage or continuation of existing policy protection with a cancer health history are frequently restrictive through increased premiums, waivers for prior health problems, and various waiting periods.

In eleven states health insurance availability is guaranteed by law to any individual unable otherwise to qualify. The major problem with this is the high cost, which runs approximately $2000 per year, for the uninsured individual who participates.

There is little uniformity among the insurance companies who write such insurance. There have been few advancements in cancer underwriting in the past decade. It is possible to use insurance brokers to shop around looking for available insurance.

Twelve states now have pooling of health insurance. The latest state to have such coverage is Illinois. Nineteen states are considering pooled insurance plans both for health insurance and comprehensive major medical insurance. Payment is provided by the individual, the insurance company, and the state. This rate may be 150 percent of the group rate but could be as low as 125 percent of the group rate. Each state has a variation on the pooled theme and the requirements for eligibility include those of state residence, prior rejection by an insurance company for health insurance, or the possession of existing health coverage that costs more than the pooled rate. High risk pools provide an economically feasible means of providing coverage when the insured would otherwise be relegated to Medicaid or Medi-Cal.

Some of us have great difficulty in interpreting the legalese of a health insurance policy. Words such as *reasonable* and *necessary* were often used in the past and seemed to be easily interpretable until refinements in health care delivery became complex and expensive. The rising cost of medical malpractice has altered the way cancer treatment is delivered and, as a result, cancer care has become much more expensive. Modern treatments, such as marrow transplants and Interleukin therapy may be outrageously expensive but are becoming more commonplace in routine cancer care and will increase the total cancer cost. The cost of delivering cancer care using the protocols of clinical trials will demand the apportionment of responsibility for payment to be split between the insurance company and a research arm. The request for insurance coverage for unproven methods of cancer treatment is an increasing problem and often results in litigation. Specialized cancer insurance policies remain an unsatisfactory purchase and are often sold to paternal groups or trade groups using fear of a dreaded disease as a way to protect the insured against such an illness. In general, they remain a poor buy with limited benefits and high cost. Most of these policies are sold under high pressure and in some states cancer insurance policies cannot be sold.

COMPENDIUM OF INSURANCE OPTIONS

If a person is not already insured, several options to seek coverage are available for the individual with a past history of cancer. An independent broker may be able to locate a reasonable benefit package; group insurance is always preferable to individual insurance. Obtaining employment is the surest way to get access to group insurance. The best type of plan is to get a guaranteed issue, one in which employees are eligible for benefits regardless of prior health history. Children of school age with cancer might be able to get coverage through school insurance. Health maintenance organizations (HMOs) often offer one period of open enrollment each year where applicants are accepted regardless of health history. Some individuals can apply for group insurance from fraternal or professional organizations and the guaranteed issue plan is preferable. One may be eligible for Medicare if under age 65 and permanently disabled, or have been receiving Social Security benefits for two years. Low income or unemployed individuals may be eligible for Medi-Cal or Medicaid. If one is currently employed, it is wise not to leave a job until the conversion options of your current plan have been explored. Legislation proposing catastrophic health insurance for individuals with illnesses such as cancer has been passed in the most recent session of Congress and is now available to those eligible for Medicare.

SUMMARY OF EMPLOYMENT ISSUES

Work is a critical component of total rehabilitation for individuals with a cancer health history. Employment provides income and financial security, access to insurance benefits, access to professional and social support, as well as a source of self-esteem. There are a growing number of cancer survivors for whom employment retains long-term significance.

There are certain individuals who have a significant potential for employment problems associated with a cancer history and these individuals would benefit from job counseling. Those at greatest risk are: blue-collar workers; low-income, seasonal, or marginally employed workers; nonwhites; young people with little or no established work experience; individuals with noted physical disabilities; those with significant treatment sequelae or advanced cancer; or individuals close to retirement age. The return to work after a cancer illness is often the outcome of successful rehabilitation and the workplace is clearly the site to demonstrate such benefits.

Some of the major job discrimination problems are denial of new employment, termination, transfers, demotion, curtailment of work, refusal to accommodate, or reduction of fringe benefits.

Rough estimates of the overall problem may be summarized as follows: About 20 percent do not return to work but 80 percent do. Of those who do return to work, somewhere between 60 percent and 85 percent have work problems and about 20 to 25 percent have new employment refusal. Job counseling and employer education are the most obvious solutions for these problems. The legislative approach is necessary but its application may be prolonged and often expensive and not always successful. A cancer patient has to have certain legal rights and certainly reasonable accommodations must be made by the employer on his return to work when necessary. Public policy needs to be focused on the plight of the cancer patient in the workplace and employers, both public and private, must get on the bandwagon to eliminate discrimination and to reintegrate all work-able persons with a health history involving cancer into the productive ranks of society.

REFERENCES

DeVita, V. Annual Report, National Cancer Institute, 1986.
Leeds, B. Personal communication, 1986.
Mor, V. Paper presented at American Cancer Society Workshop on Employability and Insurability, New Orleans, LA, December 1986.

Rice, D. P., Hodgson, T. A., & Capell, F. The economic burden of cancer, 1985. Presented at Cancer Care and Costs: DRGs and Beyond. San Diego: May 29, 1987.

Sheppard, C. Personal communication, 1986.

Subject Index

Author Index

Contributors

Ariel B. Baker
Tumor Registry
University of Kansas Medical Center
Kansas City, KS

Ivan Barofsky
Institute of Social Oncology
Silver Spring, MD

Mary J. Bartholomew
Department of Behavioral Sciences
Milton S. Hershey Medical Center
Pennsylvania State University
Hershey, PA

Joan Bloom
Department of Social and Administrative Health Sciences
School of Public Health
University of California
Berkeley, CA

Richard Cox
Department of Radiology

Division of Radiation Therapy
Stanford University Medical Center
Stanford, CA

F. L. Feldman
School of Social Work
University of Southern California
Los Angeles, CA

Patricia Fobair
Department of Radiology
Division of Radiation Therapy
Stanford University Medical Center
Stanford, CA

Patricia A. Ganz
Department of Medicine
San Fernando Valley Program
UCLA School of Medicine
Veterans Administration Medical Center
Sepulveda, CA

Ruth S. Hassanein
Department of Biometry
University of Kansas
Medical Center
Kansas City, KS

Richard L. Heinrich
Behavioral Medicine Research Laboratory
Veterans Administration Medical Center
Sepulveda, CA

Joan F. Hermann
Department of Social Services
Fox Chase Cancer Center
Philadelphia, PA

Frederick F. Holmes
Department of Medicine
University of Kansas Medical Center
Kansas City, KS

Grace Holmes

Department of Preventative Medicine and Pediatrics
University of Kansas Medical Center
Kansas City, KS

Richard Hoppe
Department of Radiology
Division of Radiation Therapy
Stanford University Medical Center
Stanford, CA

Peter S. Houts
Department of Behavioral Science
Milton S. Hershey Medical Center
Pennsylvania State University
Hershey, PA

S. Behnham Kahn
Departments of Hematology and Oncology
Hahnemann University Medical College
Philadelphia, PA

Allan Lipton
Department of Medicine
Milton S. Hershey Medical Center
Pennsylvania State University
Hershey, PA

Katherine M. Marconi
Bureau of Planning
Pennsylvania Department of Health
Harrisburg, PA

Robert J. McKenna
University of Southern California
Wilshire Oncology Medical Group
Los Angeles, CA

Cyndie Coscarelli Schag
Behavioral Medicine Research Laboratory
Veterans Administration Medical Center
Sepulveda, CA

George W. Schelzel
Division of Chronic Diseases

Pennsylvania Department of Health
Harrisburg, PA

David Spiegel
Department of Psychiatry
Stanford University Hospital
Stanford, CA

M. Jane Teta
Safety and Environmental Affairs Department
Union Carbide Corporation
Danbury, CT

Nicholas Toghia
Acret and Perochet
Los Angeles, CA

Anna Verghese
Department of Radiology
Division of Radiation Therapy
Stanford University Medical Center
Stanford, CA

Joyce M. Yasco
School of Nursing
University of Pittsburgh
Pittsburgh, PA

About the Editor

IVAN BAROFSKY is a psychologist whose career includes teaching, research, and government service. His major area of research interest is quality of life assessment, particularly of the chronically ill. He became interested in the work history of the cancer patient while working for the National Cancer Institute. He has edited or coedited four books, most recently *Rehabilitation and Treatment of the Head and Neck Cancer Patient* (with E. Meyers and J. Yates, 1986), and has published numerous research papers.